DEMENTIA DIARY

A Caregiver's Journal

By

Robert Tell

ISBN 1-4116-6577-5

Published by RTP Press

Printed in the United States of America

Website: http://www.lulu.com/DEMENTIA-DIARY

ACKNOWLEDGMENTS

I am deeply grateful to the members of the Wordsmiths (a Michigan writers group): Maria Abulnar, Ann D'Arcy, Gail Felker, Marguerite Peraino, Sharon Rocklin, and Marty Toohey, who patiently listened to me read the words, sentences, paragraphs, and chapters of this manuscript, made their suggestions, listened to my revisions, and then did it all again and again.

Thanks, too, to Tom Cranshaw, Dr. Seth Goldsmith, and Betty and Donald Bieber. They have "walked the walk" with their own loved ones and have openly shared their personal experiences with me. Their comments on my manuscript were invaluable.

I also want to express my gratitude to the wonderful professionals and volunteers whose efforts and love did so much to support my mother as she struggled with all her might to keep from losing herself to her disease.

I am indebted to the Graduate School of Public Health at Columbia University, which sensitized me as a young graduate student to the needs of the aged and the importance of creating quality facilities for long-term care in America.

One of my favorite poets, Charles Simic, needs acknowledgement as well. His essays in his book, "The Unemployed Fortune-Teller," <u>The University of Michigan Press</u>, provided the quotes for my Bookends.

Daughter Celeste, and sons Perry and Brian, deserve special recognition for the understanding and kindness they have provided during their grandmother's long decline.

Most of all, I want to thank my wife Elaine whose constant support has been a blessing and whose insights and ideas have made this a much better book.

Finally, let me acknowledge the contribution of my parents. If my father were still alive, and if my mother were not lost in her moment-to-moment world of dementia, I believe they would be pleased to have their personal story used to help others to cope with a loved one's dementia.

Dementia Diary

CONTENTS

Dementia Diary

For Mom

PREFACE

Dementia Diary

This is neither a guidebook nor compendium of advice about how to cope with caring for an aging parent or spouse with dementia. There are literally hundreds of such tomes available. My hope, instead, is that this book will become a kind of "portable support group" for caregivers.

Dementia Diary is first and foremost a memoir about what it's like to be the only child, a son, and the caregiver of a widowed and cognitively impaired mother who lives alone half a continent away.

Those who know my family will recognize that the name I've given my mother in this book, Minnie Sweet, is not her real name. Why did I change her name? I have two reasons.

First, even though the narrative is largely autobiographical, some facts have been fictionalized for effect. Second, and more important, writing this memoir has been one of the most emotionally difficult projects I have ever undertaken.

In order for me to attempt it with even a semblance of objectivity, I required an artifact. Using fabricated names was that artifact—it was a distancing technique that enabled me to approach this powerful topic with safety, compassion and humor. So all of the names in this memoir are fictitious, including my parent's and mine. This worked for me and I hope it works for you.

It is also possible that someone with one of the names I used may read this book. If so, please understand the happenstance involved, and accept my apologies. Any resemblance to any real persons living or dead is purely coincidental.

I also intend for the institutions that served my mother to remain anonymous. She was fortunate to have found her way to some wonderful facilities and programs that, I believe, extended her years and the quality of her life. However, for consistency with the "semi-fictional" nature of this memoir, these institutions are best left unidentified, and any resemblance to actual facilities and programs is purely coincidental.

A word about Mom's long, slow descent into the opaque fog of multi-infarct dementia: This is a different syndrome than the well-known dementia called Alzheimer's disease, and it can be caused by frequent "silent" mini-strokes.

Here is the way a physician described the condition to me: the "victim" of such events may not be, indeed usually is not, aware that anything out of the ordinary has occurred. Neither are his or her significant others.

Perhaps there is momentary weakness, headache, or dizziness, but nothing major. Over time, however, enough damage is done to the brain that symptoms begin to appear. While some of these manifestations are unique to this syndrome, all dementias have certain behavioral commonalities that will be recognized in these pages.

I address this book to readers who are actively involved in care giving for loved ones with dementia, to those who have had this responsibility in the past, and to those who expect to face it in the future. Perhaps you will find a nugget here and there with which to identify, and from which to draw some comfort and support.

I also address this book to professionals charged with the care of persons with dementia. Perhaps it will provide a bit of insight into the perspective of a family member attempting to understand and deal with a loved one's loss of identity, memory, and cognition.

The inspiration for this diary was a talk that I was invited to give to a conference of caregivers sponsored by an adult day care program for people with dementia. The agenda included speeches by a psychiatrist and a geriatrician, followed by a panel of four caregivers reporting on their own experiences.

The purpose was to educate, inform and support an audience of caregivers who were struggling, largely in isolation, with all sorts of issues, and to provide an opportunity for them to share experiences and to ask questions.

At first, I didn't want to make this presentation. I thought it would be an improper invasion of my mother's privacy to talk about her in a public forum. Besides, it was an emotionally powerful subject and, even though I had done a lot of public speaking, I wasn't sure I could handle this one in a calm and professional manner.

But the program sponsors prevailed. All of the other panel participants were women, they told me. They said that the program needed a man who was willing to share his experience as a caregiver, as well as his feelings. Men don't easily do this kind of thing, they said, so "please," they pleaded, and finally wore down my resistance. They pointed out that lots of men are caregivers and that these listeners would appreciate hearing a presentation by a man about this sensitive subject.

In retrospect, they were right. The male caregivers in the audience, and there were many, directed most of their questions to me, and quite a few approached me afterwards to thank me. They suggested that a book describing my experience as a male caregiver is urgently needed in the marketplace. Existing books, they said, do not address their feelings and unique responsibilities as sons and husbands.

I also asked many of the women present if such a book would find a readership among female caregivers. Interestingly, they thought it would—that women, too, would benefit from reading a man's point of view on the care giving experience.

I learned a lot that evening. The presentations and audience questions taught me that the kinds of bittersweet anecdotes described in Dementia Diary are the common lot of all who deal with the reality of dementia in a loved one.

This is a disease that knows no boundaries. It is blind to the categories in which we usually place our fellow human beings. It can occur at the age of 55 or 85. It can happen to Blacks, Whites, Hispanics, Asians, Jews, Christians, Muslims, males and females, rich and poor. It has not spared ex-presidents.

Tears are shed by husbands and wives, sons and daughters, brothers and sisters—in fact anyone responsible for the care of a loved one with dementia. I hope that this book will help all such wonderworkers to understand that they are not alone. My mother would want it that way.

In the pages that follow, her story has been deliberately paced to mimic the unhurried rhythm of her gradual slide into cognitive disability, barely perceptible on a day-to-day basis, but dramatic and frightening when viewed through my own retrospectoscope over the long term.

Some chapters, especially the early ones in the book, may not reveal Mom's (Minnie Sweet's) growing deficits to the reader. Some of the anecdotes may seem like the normal foibles of an aging woman rather than a person with a serious dementia. That's what I thought too.

It's only when we get to the later stages (or later chapters) that we can see, with hindsight and in the light of her full-blown memory impairment, that the signs and symptoms were there from the beginning.

Keep in mind, also, that the young Minnie Sweet would have been mortified by many of the attitudes and behaviors of the elderly Minnie Sweet. We would have had to explain to her, just as we ourselves had to learn, that the latter was part of the disease process, and not her true personality and character.

Finally, it is my wish that the reader will see beyond the sadness, tragedy and, yes, comedy sometimes associated with the evening hours of life, and will recognize that dementia, while terrible, does not diminish the essential humanity of the afflicted individual.

ROBERT TELL, Farmington Hills, Michigan

BOOKEND—1993

"A poem is an invitation to a voyage. As in life, we travel to see fresh sights."
—Charles Simic

It's downhill now and going fast
I don't know how long she can last
I picture her in decades past
And I deny the truth.

She was a woman smart and bright
Whose energy gave off a light
I picture her all dressed in white
And I deny the truth

Her beauty gone—her judgment lost
Her affection for me now is forced
She's terrifying when she's crossed
And I deny the truth

She's widowed now and all alone
She sets a self-destructive tone
It's hard to love this angry crone
And I deny the truth

I grieve for who she was when I
Was young and did not have to lie
So many memories to untie
And I deny the truth

The truth is that she soon may die
And then I'll have to learn to cry
And also have to face this lie
And not deny the truth

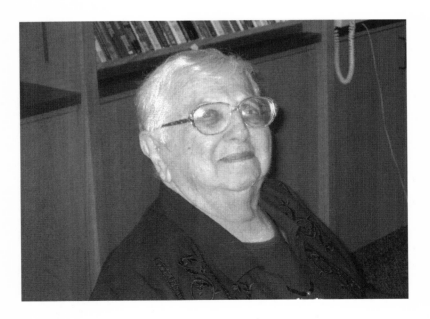

1993

Dementia Diary

WHO IS MINNIE SWEET?

Dementia Diary

My name is Jerry Sweet and it is my sweet pleasure to be sharing this story with you. That's right, Jerry Sweet—Sid and Minnie's only child. I'll be your tour guide for this entire tale.

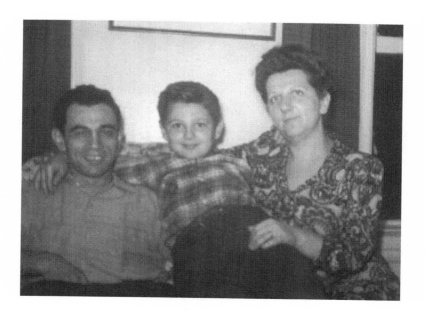

I assume, if you are reading this, that you are a caregiver or, if not, that you know someone who is. Either way, I think you will be able to relate these vignettes to your own experience and observations.

Throughout this narrative, I have tried to document the shifts in Minnie's slipping cognition. My purpose has been to demonstrate, with anecdotes and description, the various stages in her disease as it developed from its subtle beginnings to the present time.

Most of these pages track Minnie's life after the age of seventy-seven when Sidney died and her cognitive deficits were exposed. However, for you to truly appreciate the extent of the damage to this previously vital and energetic woman, you need to meet her in her younger years.

So let me introduce you to Minnie Sweet in happier days before her dementia came calling.

Minnie's history was actually rather typical. In the early 20th century, millions of immigrants from Eastern Europe could tell a similar tale. She was born in 1913, in Vilna, Lithuania, one of the three children that beat the odds and survived. Besides Minnie, there was her older sister Beverly, and a brother, Henry. Four other siblings died before reaching their first birthdays.

In spite of primitive pre-natal care, non-existent well-baby care, poverty, malnutrition, and the daily violence that permeated her world, Minnie decided to live. It was an early example of a biological hardiness that was to serve her well in the years ahead.

When Minnie was two years old, economic decline and anti-Semitic harassment in Eastern Europe were growing more serious day by day. Minnie's parents (and my grandparents), Morris and Rebecca Goldberg, decided to escape these dangers and come to America.

They arrived at Ellis Island in 1915, terrified about the possibility of being sent back by the United

States authorities. Minnie had rickets, a nutritional disease prevalent at the time among the children of the immigrant poor.

A deficiency of vitamin D and/or calcium was the cause, but it was easily corrected if caught in time. However, it affected bone growth and it was not uncommon for would-be Americans to be shipped back for this, or for even less serious health issues.

Luck was with the Goldberg's that day. They passed through the inspection easily, breathed a big sigh of relief, and settled in the Brownsville-East New York section of Brooklyn.

Other relatives also immigrated to that location, and it was fast becoming a cultural center for thousands of Jewish refugees that shared the Goldberg's history, concerns, beliefs and ethnic background.

Life was economically poor, but socially rich. Morris worked in the needle trades and Rebecca stayed home to have one more child, a girl named Charlotte, and to maintain a home for her family. Surrounded by siblings, cousins, aunts, uncles, and other family and friends, Minnie thrived. She became a real American girl. Soon the flapper years were happening, and the Great Depression was still in the future.

Attending college, or even completing high school, was a stretch for most new Americans, especially girls, back then (although Minnie did feel much pride when, decades later, she earned a GED high school equivalency diploma). Rather, it was expected that young people would work to help support the family.

And Minnie did. She became a cosmetologist and manicurist, and went to work for Mme. Sweet's Beauty Salon. It wasn't long before the boss's son,

Sidney Sweet, noticed her—much to his mother's dismay. Notwithstanding her objection to Sidney's fraternizing with the help, a romance blossomed that culminated in a marriage in 1933.

In spite of the Depression, Minnie and Sidney pursued the American dream and became a happy, optimistic couple. They were embraced lovingly by one and all—except by Mme. Sweet, who did everything she could to undermine the relationship. She eventually accepted the inevitable, but not before enabling a lifelong bitterness in her daughter-in-law, who never quite forgave her.

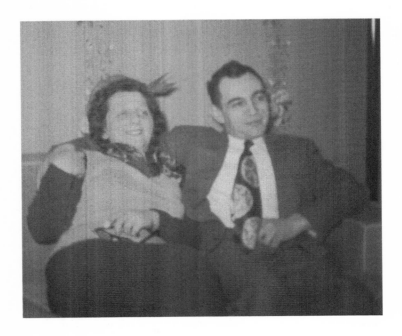

In those days, the sport of boxing was a pathway out of poverty for many immigrant young men, and fighters such as Jack Dempsey and Barney Ross were their role models. Dreaming of money and fame, Sidney Sweet decided to try his hand at prize fighting, but he soon had second thoughts when his nose was broken in the ring.

In 1937, I came along and that changed everything. As a new dad, Sidney now needed to make a steady living. So he took his squashed nose out of the ring and joined the electrician's union. Minnie became a full time mom lavishing love and attention on her only child.

In 1946, Sidney traded his blue-collar shirts for an entrepreneur's portfolio. He gave up being a master electrician in order to open a small factory for the manufacture of leather novelties.

When I was nine years old, Minnie felt free to begin her new career as the well-organized and capable foreman of the family's budding manufacturing business—and she was terrific. She was the chief operating officer of the business, the human resources department, the bookkeeper, and the detail person, while Sidney concentrated on product development, sales, and production policy. They were a great team.

So Minnie and Sidney settled into a life surrounded by warm and stable family relationships and friendships, and they began to experience some of the economic success of post-war America. They moved their home multiple times in the 1940's, 1950's and 1960's, each time into a "better" Brooklyn neighborhood. America was being good to these refugees from European poverty and hate, and their patriotic feelings were very strong.

As the economy of the late 1960's overheated, it ultimately reached the working and lower middle classes. It seemed to the Sweets that everyone they

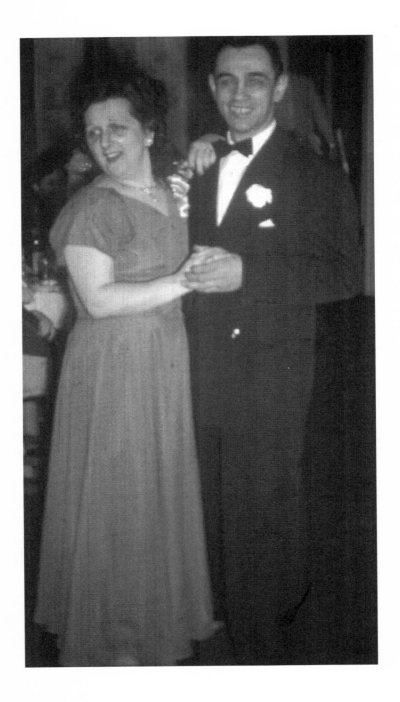

knew had great investments and a winter home in Florida, and they wanted onto this bandwagon.

Minnie and Sidney began "snow birding" to Southeastern Florida in the late 1960's to see if they might like it. It didn't take long for them to become property owners and permanent residents in this fast developing region.

Now Minnie really came into her own. She began to apply her considerable organizational skills to various non-profit leadership activities in New York and in Florida. She discovered a love and a talent for communal affairs and accepted one assignment after another.

Matron of the Eastern Star; founder and president of at least three Hadassah chapters; member of the town's library board and its Director of Volunteers; leadership roles in B'nai Brith Women and Jewish War Veterans—and these are just for starters. It was these organizations that supplied the deep and lasting friendships that blessed Minnie and Sidney for the several decades of their lives in Florida.

Of course, the idyll I've been describing had to end. Even as Minnie multi-tasked and spread her social wings across Southeastern Florida, something was changing in her brain and personality. That something was mistakenly assumed by those closest to her to be excessive stubbornness and selfishness. We were right in what we observed, but wrong about the cause.

In 1990, Sidney died and Minnie's descent down the "slippery slope" of multi-infarct dementia accelerated. Today, in 2005, she has not yet reached the base of this slope, but she is certainly nearing the end of her journey.

At first, when she was beginning her slide, none of her loved ones, including me (especially me), understood that her sometimes difficult and abrasive behavior was part of a progressive disease process.

Today, her illness is obvious. Looking back, milestones in her decline can be identified. The various chapters of this book are intended to give life to the circumstances surrounding these turning points.

At each of her transitions, whenever Minnie reached a new low in functioning, I thought that she could not decline further and still remain "alive." Each time, it was like a mini-death. Each time, I grieved anew.

Often, just when I had finally made my peace with her new level, she would rally and seem to regain ground that she had lost. When this occurred, I usually allowed myself to be duped into believing that she was not as bad as I had feared. Each time, though, something soon happened to highlight Minnie's new deficits.

Whenever I thought that she could not possibly lose additional cognition and continue to function as a viable human being, it turned out that she had not yet reached bottom. It seems that there is no conclusion to the deterioration process, other than the grave.

As I write this, Minnie is getting ready to experience her ninety-second birthday. No one close to her ever expected her to live so long. That she did so is both a blessing and a curse. For her more than for me.

Dramatic changes took place in her in the years since Sidney died, changes that became more noticeable and more frequent over time. She gradually became mild and amiable, non-confrontational, and unlike the agitated Minnie that emerged from mourning her husband's death.

Observing these changes in the early stages of her dementia, I was forced to marvel: is this the mother who made me crazy all those years when her emotions were out of control? Or is this gentle and loving paragon of a happy old age the true, underlying person?

Did the psychotropic drugs she took mask her authentic nature or, conversely, did these medications permit the real, kind, and thoughtful Minnie to shine through at last? To what extent is personality only chemistry? Who is the real Minnie Sweet?

In 1997, Minnie moved up north to be near family. Thankfully, she is still among us. Of course, no one knows know how much time she has left and, as she said long ago, she has "longevity." Every day that goes by, however, sees further diminution in her capabilities.

When she first came to live near me, I visited several times a week for an hour or so and, whenever possible, took her out of the institutional environment. Later, when I could no longer take her on outings, she could still reminisce, share memories, look at family photos, sit outside in nice weather, and maintain a reasonable conversation.

Even the telephone was a useful medium for staying in touch. Today, our phone conversations are no more, and my visits have become less frequent and shorter. She is thrilled when she sees me and, remarkably, still knows who I am.

Occasionally, she will respond to my questions with one-word answers. More frequently, she says nothing. If I stop talking, we sit in silence. Soon, with me holding her hand, she falls asleep in her wheelchair.

Yet, until recently, Minnie kept radiating love and happiness. She sometimes still does, although less often these days. Does her life have quality? Who can say?

Before she came up north, I would have argued that no one in her current condition could enjoy life. I would have said that I'd never want to live in such circumstances. Today, I'm not so sure.

Every moment of every day is new to Minnie Sweet. She still smiles a lot. Her dentures are frequently missing or lost and, like an infant, she shows a lot of gums—but she's quick to smile...and she still blows kisses to everyone.

Quality of life? What is that? Whatever it is, for most of her time here, I think Minnie had it.

SOME ARE CALLED

One Sunday morning in December 1990, I was enjoying the quiet isolation of my business office while trying to clean up the loose ends of a hectic workweek. No one was around and I was sailing along, making great progress.

I was feeling particularly happy. Business was booming. Several new contracts had been faxed in late Friday afternoon, accounts receivable were up to date, major projects were moving well toward completion, and I was beginning to think about heading home.

"Ring." It was the phone. It didn't actually ring but, instead, made that bone jarring electronic sound that has replaced the mechanical bell of older telephones (When did that triumph of 21st Century technology occur?). There is no word yet invented in the English language to adequately describe that sound. So...

"Ring," will have to do.

It took me several moments to react. After all, who could be calling a business office on a Sunday morning? It must be a wrong number, I thought. I didn't expect my wife, Nadine, to call. She knew that I preferred to work undisturbed on weekend office visits. I debated not answering it, but the so-called ring was persistent and, finally, as much from curiosity as anything else, I gave in.

"Hello?"

"Jerry?" It was Nadine's voice.

I decided to be flippant. "You were expecting, maybe, Woody Allen?" I quipped, to let her know that I didn't mind the interruption. "What's up?"

The first sign of trouble was the silence at the other end. It was only a moment, but it was long enough to send me a signal. Whatever it was, Nadine was either reluctant to say, or else she did not know quite how to proceed.

"Jerry, I'm sorry to bother you. I know how much you..."

"It's Okay, Nadine. I'm almost done for today. I was just wrapping up. I'll be home in half an hour."

"Oh," and then silence for another interminable moment. Then, "Listen. It can wait. Just come home."

All my antennae were up now. "Nadine," I said. "I've got a minute. You called for a reason. So now I'm curious. What's happening?"

"Really, Jerry, it can wait. If I knew you were getting ready to leave, I wouldn't have called."

Now I was getting alarmed or annoyed. I wasn't really sure which. Probably both. There was something in Nadine's voice that scared me.

"What's with all the mystery?" I asked. "Don't make me crazy. You called me, so what is it that couldn't wait before; and, now, all of a sudden, it can?"

"Your Aunt Charlotte called."

This was my mother Minnie's younger sister, my favorite Aunt, and the closest thing I had to a sibling. She called frequently, but not usually on Sunday mornings.

I didn't know the details yet, but I was beginning to guess where this conversation was going. Hoping that I was jumping to false conclusions, I asked,

"Charlotte? What did she want? Is everything Okay in Florida?"

"She just called and asked me to contact you and ask you to come home."

This was getting stranger and stranger. I was starting to understand how a district attorney must feel when cross-examining a hostile witness.

My poor wife was clearly in distress. I was not yet completely conscious of the fact that what she had to say would hurt me, but my instincts were figuring it out fast.

"Nadine, come clean," I begged. "Why did she ask you to do this?"

"She asked me not to tell you on the phone. She just said to get you to come home as soon as possible."

Bingo! Minnie had been ailing recently with chronic obstructive pulmonary disease, congestive heart failure, anxiety attacks and depression, high blood pressure, and spinal arthritis.

So now I thought I knew why Nadine was calling. We had often discussed the relative issues associated with the loss of either of my parents in terms of who might go first. Minnie always seemed to be the more fragile of the two, so I was quite sure of the answer when I asked quietly, holding my breath.

"It's my mother, isn't it?"

"No."

Oh, oh. That didn't leave a lot of alternatives. Still, I asked, hoping for another negative, "My father?"

"Yes."

Pause.

"Dead?" Please God, have her say "No."

"Yes."

The room began to spin. I said nothing. I couldn't speak. I just sat there holding the receiver. From somewhere deep inside a tremor started and worked its way outward gathering momentum as it migrated. Soon it was forcing its way up through my chest and out through my throat. A huge sob broke forth surprising me with its power.

"Are you alright?" Nadine asked, her voice barely a whisper.

"No," I replied. I wanted to say more but choked on my words. I just sat there and tried to fight the sobs, but it was impossible. They consumed me. Nadine sat patiently on the other end, saying nothing, waiting for my lead. Finally, when the spasm ended, I asked,

"How?"

She filled me in on what Charlotte had told her.

"Sears?" I repeated.

"Sears," she said again.

"Returning a rug?" I repeated. I had heard her, but it was a comic twist to a personal tragedy, and very hard to absorb.

"Returning a rug," she repeated, and both of us started to laugh. In between the tears, we laughed until it hurt. Feeling guilty about the levity, but unable to ignore the irony in the situation, I laughed until I cried. Then, emotionally spent, I said,

"How's Minnie taking it? Did Charlotte say?"

"Not good. She's at Charlotte's apartment. Charlotte says she was crying hysterically, but she's sleeping now."

Another deep breath. It was hard for me to talk. "Call the airlines," I managed to croak out.

"It's done. We have a 9:05 am flight tomorrow. I've called the kids too. They're all planning to go."

I shook my head to try to clear it. "It's all happening so fast. I can't believe he's dead."

No response from Nadine for a moment. Then, "So, are you coming home now?"

I nodded, although there was no one that could see me. "I'll be home in twenty minutes," I said.

"Will you be okay?" she asked.

"I think so. Listen, did you really believe you could get me home without telling me the truth?"

"It seems pretty silly now," Nadine replied. "Charlotte was insistent that I shouldn't say anything on the phone, that I had to get you home one way or another first. It seemed like a good idea at the time."

"Nice try!" I said. "See ya soon."

DYING TO SHOP

When Minnie and Sidney Sweet retired to Florida around 1970, he was in his mid 60's and she in her late 50's. They were young retirees. Sid sold his small manufacturing business, and the building housing it, for just enough money to promise a comfortable, if not opulent, lifestyle.

So they took the plunge. They left their only son. They left their daughter-in-law, and their three grandchildren. They left siblings, cousins and lifelong friends, and they bought a condo in a Florida retirement village.

You know the kind. Two bedrooms. Two bathrooms. A living room leading to a Florida room (porch, to you) that looked out at the seventh hole. A small kitchen (who cooks? It's cheaper to eat out with the Early Bird)—and insufficient closet space.

The community boasted a full time resort atmosphere complete with clubhouse, swimming pools, tennis courts, golf course, transit system, and security gate. And, of course, shuffleboard. The ubiquitous shuffleboard. The Sweets never looked back!

The stock market decline of the 1970's took the glow off the carefree nature of their relocation. It was a disappointment for Sidney, and one that attacked his self-image as a provider and protector of his family.

Even though he had no personal control over what was happening to the economy, nothing could convince him that their troubles weren't his fault. For Minnie, it was a shock to her sense of security. Her verbal expressions of these feelings did little to help Sidney overcome his guilt feelings.

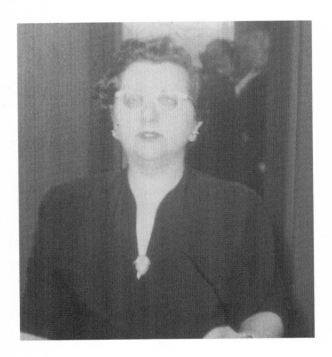

Still, the Sweets had enough money left, when combined with Social Security and Medicare, to maintain a modest but adequate existence. So they survived. Actually, they thrived. In spite of the economy, they soared. The years flew by. They joined every charitable organization they could find. So did all the other newcomers.

The Sweets were warm and affable people. They provided a happy home for me as a youngster and, after I married, a loving embrace for the new family that I was creating.

It was not surprising that they made many new friends in Florida. People liked and respected them. Sidney's sense of humor and his integrity were widely admired, and he was a role model that many aspired to imitate. This was especially true for his son.

Minnie's enthusiastic and outgoing nature attracted people to her like bears to honey. They played golf, went to meetings, played golf, enjoyed social events, played golf, had doctor appointments (of which there were many), played golf and, of course, they shopped.

Shopping, for most of us, is about meeting our basic needs and desires for food, clothing, gadgets and luxury items. For some people, however, it has other satisfactions and it fills other needs.

It may be a social event with emotional overtones—or a way to fill time in an otherwise boring life—or even, for some, an addiction that brings cheer to an otherwise dreary disposition. This can be as true for snowbirds and retirees of the Sunbelt as it is for the rest of the population—maybe even truer.

Consider a typical day in the life of the Sweets. In the morning they'd shop for, say, a toaster oven. They'd buy one, take it home and plug it in. They'd then enjoy a nice lunch with slices of toast made in their new purchase.

But there'd be a problem. The bread might be browning less evenly than expected. Maybe it would even be getting a little too dark and crisp along the edges. They wanted a perfect piece of toast, something that the new oven seemed incapable of producing.

Too bad! They'd have to bring the toaster back. They'd return it to the store for a refund and then, of course, would proceed to buy something else that would probably have to be returned the next day. And so it went. Day after day after day.

And the Sweets were joined in these daily shopping adventures by thousands of their contemporaries. One wonders how the retailers managed to stay in business.

If this description seems amusing, consider the other side of the story. Shopping can provide a brief escape from the preoccupation with death and disease that is the constant companion of the seniors that populate these retirement communities.

Their adult children "up north" may still believe in the illusion of their own immortality, but our shoppers know better. And yet, these older Americans somehow manage to mix a laugh or two with the bad things that happen daily to their neighbors, friends, and to themselves. It's how they cope with their reality.

A case in point: While there isn't anything happy in the tragedy about to be described, there is a bit of the ironic. Something that may elicit a smile or two even as it evokes the tears. Here's what happened.

One day in 1990, Minnie and Sidney Sweet decided to go to a nearby Sears & Roebuck store. It was early and the store just opened. They entered the store and, as they walked toward the escalators, Sidney died. That's right, he died. On the spot.

One minute he was walking alongside Minnie and the next he was laying face down where he had pitched forward onto the floor. With no sound, no cry of pain, nothing. His complexion was grey, and he was gone.

Later, a doctor was to say it was a massive heart event, that Sidney had felt no discomfort and never knew what happened. The doctor said it was a good way to die, easy on the deceased, but hard on his loved ones. It was indeed very hard on his son (and I should know), but it was hardest on Minnie.

Imagine her horror. She had spent all of her married life almost totally dependent on her husband. She didn't drive (more about that at another time), was rarely separated from him, and drew her emotional strength and most of her identity from him. It was not an uncommon role for women of her generation.

Also, her dementia had started. Not that anyone close to her, or she herself, recognized that her exaggerated personality quirks and her growing memory lapses were due to illness. They were just "Minnie," and what could you do?

Perhaps Sidney knew something was amiss. Perhaps not. But without him to "cover" for her behavioral idiosyncrasies, she would become more and more exposed.

In any event, Minnie never really expected to have to face life without Sidney. Oh, she knew that they were getting into the dangerous years, and they had even talked about it. But that was an abstraction, not something that could really happen. Until that morning at Sears, when it did.

And what a way to have to face it. Alone among strangers, in a department store, sudden death. A catastrophe. She screamed and cried and couldn't be consoled. She was seventy-seven.

Why, you ask, were they in a Sears store that morning? You guessed it. They were returning a small rug they had purchased the day before for the floor of their bathroom. It didn't look as nice as they had anticipated.

Twelve years after the event, at eighty-nine, Minnie would smile when asked whether Sid died before or after they returned the rug, and whether they were able to get their refund. She would chuckle at the thought, but could not recall the answer.

A year later, at ninety, she would struggle to remember who Sidney was—and she would ask the visitor to tell her how her husband died.

SHOPPING TO DIE

There is a product that is very popular among shoppers in South Florida. It is free from the pattern of "buy today and return tomorrow" that was described in the previous chapter. This product is known euphemistically as "Pre-Need."

It is sold by funeral directors, of which there are very many. Retirement communities breed undertakers and cemeteries in the same way that young family suburbs grow childcare centers and elementary schools.

Morticians have discovered an undeniable truth about merchandising their wares. It is very difficult to return a cemetery plot or coffin, especially after it has been used. This gives the death business an advantage that has to be the envy of merchants selling more mundane wares.

So what, exactly, is Pre-Need? The idea, which is attractive to many retirees, is that they can make decisions concerning their deaths while still alive and vigorous.

Purchasers of Pre-Need packages hope that all will go smoothly when they die, and that they will be sparing their loved ones the turmoil and trauma of having to make all sorts of tough choices under time and emotional pressures.

By arranging all of these things, and paying for them in advance, the theory goes, the temptation to buy the most expensive casket and services (because nothing is too good for "Dad") can be avoided.

The cynical view is that Pre-Need is a clever scheme that greedy funeral parlor owners have invented to lock in their customers, and to obtain up-front capital on which to earn interest. They sell the "product," usually on an installment contract basis, with high, if not usurious, interest rates.

The buyer thus loses the investment interest that would have been earned by the dollars spent on the Pre-Need contract. It is the mortician that now earns the investment interest—and, to make the deal even sweeter, the buyer gets to pay credit interest to the mortician for the privilege of deferring final payment.

Not bad (for the funeral parlor, that is)!

In addition, the mortician is assured that the mortuary's investment for cemetery land is quickly returned to the business, along with a nice margin of profit, long before it's actually needed for the purpose for which its sold. No wonder so many entrepreneurs are dying to get into this business.

The truth is that Pre-Need can be a win-win in many situations. If the funeral parlor and cemetery deliver what is promised in the contract; if they don't use the moments after death to impose the old "bait and switch" technique on guilt ridden survivors in an effort to sell higher priced product than chosen by the deceased; and if the terms of a fair and honorable agreement reached with the deceased long before the moment of need are observed, then the Pre-Need agreement may actually provide a bona fide value to the purchaser and to his or her loved ones; and a reasonable and fair business profit to the seller as well.

It is the ultimate layaway plan!

What does all this have to do with Minnie and Sidney Sweet? I'll tell you, although I'm sure that you have made the connection. Yep! The Sweets had purchased Pre-Need contracts from the Menorah Maven Funeral Home and Twilight Gardens (MMFHTG).

They were very proud of their new real estate, and felt the Pre-Need process to be an unselfish gift to their surviving family members. In fact, they seemed to enjoy taking me along on visits to the cemetery plots whenever the opportunity allowed.

Somehow, I did not find this activity to be as fun-filled as a trip to the beach but, since Dad was so excited about it, I shrugged and played along. Sidney loved to point out the aesthetics of the place.

There were no large, vertical stone markers. All graves had tasteful flat marble plaques engraved with the names of the deceased, dates of birth and death, and a few loving words. Nothing else. Rich or poor, man or woman, none had visible symbols to display worldly success or failure.

The only other option was a mausoleum-like structure that, for a price premium, would store one's remains above ground in a kind of huge, bureau-like, concrete facility.

Minnie liked that idea, but Sidney did not. He said it would be like lying between the sock drawer and the underwear. Sidney prevailed.

And so, shortly after the incident at Sears, the Sweet clan and its remaining friends gathered at MMFHTG to pay their last respects to Sidney. Minnie was still in shock and denial.

Part of her was her old well-organized self. She threw herself into coordinating the funeral arrangements with the same efficiency and energy she used to organize the three new Hadassah chapters that she subsequently served as President. This part of her persona locked her fear and anxiety up in a safe and walled compartment somewhere inside her heart and soul. She functioned, but as in a dream.

Another part of her knew, though, that this was different, that the funeral was about Sidney, and that this event was the prelude to a new life of loneliness and confusion that awaited her.

The changes that Minnie was experiencing must have frightened and worried her. For the past few years, her highs had become much too high, her lows were severe and self-destructive, and she surely felt a loss of control.

She began to malign life-long friends and family members for hurts both real and imagined. Even siblings were not excluded from her wrath. Neither was her only son. Minor affronts became major issues.

"Ma," I asked following an incident in which she was especially rude to her sister, "Why did you treat Charlotte so badly? She's been so supportive of us during this mourning period, so sensitive and kind."

"What do you mean 'us'?" Minnie answered with fire in her eyes.

"I mean you and me, Mom. I'm talking about our loss."

"In the first place, I can treat anyone any way I like. I'VE lost my husband and I'm entitled to grieve."

"Yes, but grieving doesn't give us license to be unpleasant to people, especially those who love us and wish us well."

"Again with the 'us.' I'm the one who lost my husband, so everyone can just get off my back."

"I understand that you lost your husband, Ma, but I had a loss too. I lost my Dad."

She looked stunned at this realization. "Yes," she allowed. "I guess you did. But it's not the same thing. I loved Sidney. What will I do without him?"

"I loved him too, Ma. I miss him terribly already…"

"Okay, okay, but you'll get over it. I won't."

Minnie expressed her bitterness and resentment freely and loudly to anyone who would listen, and to many who tried not to. Her world was shrinking, and she was becoming more and more isolated. Those she offended saw only a difficult personality getting worse.

No one suspected the demon growing inside of her, the illness that had begun to twist her memories, her judgment, and her emotions.

Only Sidney, who was also bewildered by the behavior of his Minnie, had been able to contain her, to do damage control and to keep the peace. He'd been shielding her. Now he was gone.

At the funeral home, Sidney lay in a partly open casket with a split lid. For a brief period prior to the service, in a departure from an ethnic tradition of closed casket funerals, his head and shoulders were visible. To my surprise, Minnie specifically requested this arrangement.

This is where I came in. Entering the visitation room prior to the service, I had a strong approach-avoidance reaction. I wanted to remember Dad as he was when he was alive and smacking golf balls into the distance at the local driving range. I did not really want to see his corpse. Yet, I couldn't turn away.

The last time I saw him alive was six months earlier at my home in the north. It was a remarkable visit, during which we talked about life and death, and about things in his past that he never opened up about before.

He cried and hugged, both of which were quite untypical behavior for him, and we shared a moment of closeness and a bond that surpassed anything previously felt between us.

At last, I thought, he is softening about his childhood. I had high hopes of finally learning the mysteries of his past that were heretofore forbidden to me. Now, that opportunity was forever gone, and his secrets were gone with him.

I approached his casket cautiously. His olive complexion, darkened further by years in the Florida sun, seemed somehow unnatural when contrasted against the clean white fabric of the casket interior. There was tightness in my abdomen as I studied him.

I held my breath and took a long, slow, painful, final look at my favorite father, my hero and my role model; and, so help me, he winked at me.

No one saw it but me. I know you think I imagined it, but I don't care. Maybe I just knew that that's what he would have done if he were capable of it. It doesn't matter. As far as I was concerned, he did it. He winked at me.

As I retreated from his casket-side, my mother, Minnie, and a "Suit" accosted me at the exit from the visitation room. I don't know how else to describe the short, very thin and pale man standing beside her. All I saw was a dark and shiny polyester suit.

The man introduced himself as the manager of the funeral home and insisted that Mom and I join him immediately in his office. I didn't know what he wanted and, frankly, at the moment I did not particularly care.

"Not right now," I resisted. "We're in mourning. What's this about?"

"It really can't wait," he persisted, "and I'm afraid that we can't continue the funeral until we sit down and talk."

Something about his words and tone told me that this was about money. He could not have chosen a more sensitive time to engage in such an insensitive demand. It was hard to contain the anger I was feeling, but I had no choice.

Mom and I followed him meekly into his office, while the funeral was placed on hold. I hoped the interruption would be short and that nobody "outside" would notice. When we were seated at a small table in his office, the Suit began to speak.

He wasn't rude. In fact he was unctuous. He got right to the point. "Your mother owes us $2200." He said. "I'm sorry, but we must have a check right now in order for our services to continue."

"They have a Pre-Need agreement with you," I said. "My understanding is that everything has been paid for."

Mom looked sheepish. The Suit cleared his throat. "Yes, they do have Pre-Need with us. That's why the balance is so low."

"Why is there a balance at all?" I asked, still confused by the shakedown I was getting.

"Let me show you," he replied, putting a stack of pink and yellow papers, invoices, and contracts on the table in front of us.

It seems that Dad had been paying out the agreement on a time contract and, when he died, there was still a balance of about $500. To that amount another $1000 had to be added for the very best coffin the funeral parlor had in its inventory. Mom had upgraded to that model today.

Then there was the extra limousine service, and on and on and on, numerous services over and above the Pre-Need arrangements, and all ordered by Minnie during the past 24 hours. The new total came to $2200. Was I prepared to write a check?

"Can't this wait until after the funeral?" I asked, hoping to have a chance to talk to my mother privately, and hoping she would write the check. She could afford it. But she was sitting silently, staring at the floor.

"I think this is in very bad taste," I said. "If we owe you some money, you'll be paid. What's the hurry now? Let's get the funeral going."

"You don't understand," said the Suit. "This is a business, and we often get stuck with bad debts. Our policy now is to collect everything that's owed in advance. I'm sorry, but no money, no more funeral today.

"You can't just stop it now," I snapped. "My father is out there lying in one of your Cadillac caskets."

"We can and we will," came the reply. "Your father can be refrigerated until the bill is paid and then we can proceed."

I couldn't believe my ears. Refrigerated! "You would really send all those mourners home at this point," I said, more as a statement then a question.

"I'm sorry. Without a check for $2200 I'd have no other choice."

Minnie looked up at me. There was a bewildered look in her eyes. She said nothing, but she did not have to. It was clear what I had to do.

"Whom do I make it out to?" I asked, taking out my pen.

DRIVING AWAY THE BLUES

Sidney never let Minnie drive. Oh, when they were younger, Minnie got her license and, occasionally, did get behind the wheel. For decades, however, Sidney just obstructed any effort to get her to drive. Every once in awhile, she would launch a mild protest.

"He won't let me drive," she would say meekly.

"What do you mean 'let you'?" I'd ask. "You're a grown woman. If you want to drive, take the keys and do it. I bet Dad won't stop you if you really insist."

"No," she'd say quietly, "He won't let me."

And that was that. Actually, she had little incentive to force the issue. For one thing, with nary a protest or complaint, Sidney drove Minnie everywhere she had to go. For another, he usually wanted to accompany her to 95% of the places where she wanted to go. So what was the big deal?

This drove Nadine and me nuts. We understood that Mom was of an immigrant generation that encouraged wives to become totally dependent on their husbands. Women had been liberated, however. Hadn't she noticed? Why didn't she demand equality with respect to driving, we asked each other? Didn't she care about her rights, we wondered?

Apparently not. It seemed that the issue was more of a problem in our minds than in Minnie or Sid's, and so we backed off. That is, while Sidney was alive and in the driver's seat, so to speak.

When Sid died, Nadine and I smelled an opportunity. Mom had lost her full time chauffer. She was going to become locationally challenged unless she moved quickly to do one of two things, or perhaps both.

One possibility was for her to utilize a local van service for seniors, a commercial taxi company, or one of the private chauffer services offered by some of the retired men in the community. The second idea involved Minnie's return to the world of car and driver. Nadine and I were aggressively pushing the latter. We would live to regret this.

It did not take much to get Minnie to acquiesce to our encouragement. She began driving Sid's Bonneville within weeks of his death. I call it Sid's Bonneville because that's what it was. He loved that car. When he wanted to buy it, he lobbied Minnie ceaselessly for months in order to gain her agreement about the expenditure.

Money had become relatively tight. "I'd like to get one more car before I die," he'd say.

"You're not dying so fast," she'd reply. "There's nothing wrong with the Buick."

"This will be my last new car," he'd come back, playing on her sympathy.

"Stop it," she'd snort. "You're breaking my heart, old man. You have at least three new cars left in you."

Well, he wore her down. Little did either really expect his words to become so prophetic. Within two years, he was dead, and Minnie was trying to pilot a car around Retiree Realm that was at least two sizes too big.

She wasn't the worst or most dangerous driver out there on the road. Countless other cognitively or physically impaired people terrorized their neighborhoods with their OPC's. Nevertheless, she was certainly holding her own.

By the way, an OPC, I'm told by my children's' generation, is an "Old Person's Car," usually a dated, extra large, GM, Ford, or Chrysler product.

Here's what happened. A few days after the funeral, Minnie needed groceries and faced her moment of truth. Call a cab or drive? It was a "no-brainer." Off she went and within a month we knew why Sidney had kept her solidly planted in the passenger seat.

First, it was the fender bender phantom.

"Ma," I asked when I'd came for a visit, "what happened to the tail light?"

"What do you mean?"

"Come look."

"Oh yeah, it's smashed. I forgot."

"How did it happen?"

"It was parked in the Publix parking lot. I noticed the damage when I got back with my groceries."

"What about the dent in the right passenger side fender?"

"These parking lots are trouble. That was when I parked near the Eckerd's drug store."

"Did you see who did it?"

Silence. Then a guilty look. Then, "No. The drivers down here are awful."

There was no point in quizzing her about the loose and hanging chrome strip, the deep scratch in the driver side door, or a half dozen other minor injuries. It was always the fender bender phantom. She saw no evil, heard no evil, and smelled no evil.

Then there was the tale of the "nice policeman."

Ring, ring. "Hello," I said.

"It's me honey. I want to tell you about the sweet officer that stopped me yesterday." Minnie laughed as she announced this as though it was the funniest thing since Milton Berle. Did I really want to know what came next? No, not really but…

"What about the sweet officer?" I asked fearing the worst.

"Well, ha, ha ha, he was so nice. He stopped me and told me I was going the wrong way on a one way street."

"What!" I yelled, blood pressure rising, "That's very dangerous, Ma. Did he give you a ticket?"

"No, of course not, silly. He knows me. This isn't the first time it's happened."

Again, "What!" I tried, and failed, to sound calm. "You're telling me it's happened before?"

"Only a couple of times. Why are you so excited?"

"Ma, it's very dangerous. You could have had a head-on. What did the policeman do?"

"I told you. He's my friend. He did what he always does."

"Which is?"

"He had me turn the car around and he told me to be more careful. He smiled, too. He's such a nice young policeman."

"He turned you around, smiled and sent you on your way? No warnings? No punishments?"

"What are you going on about? Nobody's hurt. I thought it was funny. I just wanted you to know."

"Goodbye, Ma."

"'Bye."

So much for women's lib. Seems we had created a monster and had to face the tricky task of somehow reversing course. How? That's another story.

HCFA HELPER

When Patti burst in, I was already going crazy.

The day had been wild with phone calls and I was hours behind. Stacks of pink message slips peppered my desk. Most had the boxes, "Please Call back" and "Urgent," checked off. I tried to arrange them by priority, but to no avail. As soon as I had them sorted, another call would come in demanding attention.

It had not been a pleasant day. For some reason people were short tempered and angry. Maybe it was the full moon. Who knows? Anyway, clients were growling, canceling business, hanging up on me, whatever. I had had it.

"What is it, Patti?" I snapped. "You know what my day's been like. Whatever it is, whoever it is, tell 'em I've gone to Alaska."

One of the things I like best about Patti Farmer is her even temper. No matter how agitated I become, and agitated is one of my frequent states, she offsets it with her calm and relaxed manner. I never know for sure what she's feeling. She can be dealing with inner turmoil, but you'd never know it. She's the perfect Office Manager, at least for an office like mine.

As usual, on the day in question, she ignored my abrasive words and said, "This sounds important boss. It's someone from Hickfa."

Hickfa, or HCFA was the United States Health Care Finance Administration, the agency responsible for Medicare and Medicaid, among other things.

"Oh," I said, more quietly now, wondering what they could possibly want with me. In my past life as a health policy wonk, I knew people at HCFA. Perhaps this was a blast from the past, an old colleague with something nice to say. God knows, I needed something nice that day.

"Who is it?" I asked.

"I just told you, HCFA."

"No. I mean who? What's the caller's name?"

Patti gave me a name I did not recognize. Still, I was happy for the excuse to put aside the bad news business calls and seek this change of pace.

"OK, Patti, you win," I said. "Put him through."

The voice on the phone was officious and authoritative, not at all the hoped for sound of a former colleague. This was going to be an interaction with the bureaucracy. I could tell that immediately.

"Mr. Sweet?" it said.

"Yes."

"Mr. Jerry Sweet?"

"That's me." Oh, oh! I felt my defenses rising. Maybe I should have stuck with the client callbacks.

"Are you Minnie Sweet's son?"

What now, I thought? What has Mom done now? A sense of dread washed over me. Did I need this today? What could I do? The price of being an only child is the joy of handling an elderly widowed parent with dementia. I was trapped.

"I'm her son," I replied.

"Oh, good. Listen, are you aware that your mother has switched membership in her HMO's seven times in the last twelve months?"

Oh boy, an ally, I thought, not knowing whether to laugh or to cry. During the past few years, one of Mom's lifetime patterns had become exaggerated. For as long as I could remember, she had put people on pedestals where they could do no wrong.

Inevitably, they would do something to fall off that pedestal and, as far as Mom was concerned, forever after they could do no right. This was true for friends, relatives and, of course, her professionals.

She changed doctors as often as a fashion model changed outfits. She had not had continuity in her medical care for years. It was a major worry. But changing HMO's as frequently as she had switched individual practitioners? This was a new one.

I felt glad that HCFA had caught her. I didn't know what the penalty would be, for I was certain that that's what this call was about. Mom was to be punished for abusing the system and running up its costs. That would give me the handle I needed to take control of her care.

So I said, hopefully, "I did not know, but I'm awfully glad you called."

I then unloaded all of my fears and concerns, positive that the caller would assist me with reaching my goal. After all, wasn't HCFA concerned about the proper use of the Medicare Health Maintenance Organization system?

"Listen. I understand what you're telling me," said HCFA, "but there's nothing we can do about that."

My heart sank. "So why are you calling me?" I was beginning to get irritated.

"This is the Medicare fraud division. Three of the seven changes she made were back into the Foilsick HMO. Here's what I need to know. Did your mother switch HMO's on her own initiative, or did a salesman induce her to switch."

I suddenly recalled Mom reciting the fabulous attributes of an HMO sales agent. At the time, I only half listened to this latest in a long line of pedestal dwellers. Hoo boy! I should have been paying better attention.

"I have to be truthful," I said. "I believe my mother initiated the changes herself."

"OK," said HCFA. "I'm sorry to have bothered you. That's all I needed to know."

"Wait a minute," I protested. "Aren't you gonna help me stop her from continuing this self-destructive behavior?"

"Sorry, no," came the reply. "That's not my division. Thanks for your help."

"Not your division?" I shouted. "Don't you care about...hello? Hello?"

But he was gone.

MOVED TO TEARS

For most of their lives, Sidney and Minnie Sweet liked to move. I don't mean their bodies. I mean their belongings. It was a pattern they seemed to enjoy. Between 1933 and 1971, without leaving Brooklyn, they changed residences on the average of every five years.

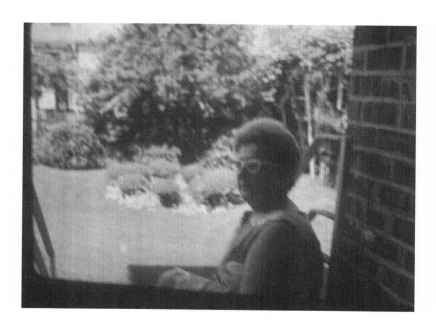

It was the same when they retired to the sunny and humid air of Southeastern Florida. They had barely settled into their first "seniors" condo when they became dissatisfied and moved again.

Then, hard to believe, they settled down at last and stopped the packing and unpacking that had so frequently punctuated their lives. They selected a brand new retiree development with hundreds of cute, look alike, detached, ranch houses. Although they did not know it at the time, this would be the last of their many homes that they would share together.

Remarkably, they seemed content with their newfound stability. Perhaps it was the executive golf course down the street, or the community clubhouse, a mere thirty-five yards from their front door, with its pool and pool tables, shuffleboard courts, card rooms, and social hall. Or, perhaps, they were finally just tired of the constant change.

Whatever the reason, the nomad pattern was deeply ingrained in Minnie and, when Sidney died, it resurfaced again. Big time! Only now the moving urge was complicated by something else. That "something" was the growing evidence that Minnie wasn't coping well.

Of course, it was understandable that continuing to live in "that" house would disturb her, with its memories of the great love of her life in every corner— but she never said so and, in fact, she denied it. On the other hand, she had lived in the same house for twenty years. A new record. It was time. Here's what she said about it:

"The neighborhood is changing."

"What do you mean, changing, Ma? It looks the same to me.

"The houses are being bought by a lower class. Every time someone moves out, the new people are not up to the standard."

"What does that mean, Ma…'not up to the standard'?"

"Just take a look up the street. Drive around. You'll see."

"I did that already. You told me to do that yesterday. The people looked nice."

"You can't tell by just looking. You have to live here to know."

"But you said I could tell by looking."

"Just forget about it, Jerry. You don't understand. I think I should sell the house."

"Is it Dad, Ma? Are you depressed living in the house you shared with him?"

"Don't be ridiculous! It's the people. I don't like the people."

This line of communication was clearly unproductive but, for a time, Minnie backed off her itch to move and seemed to become more content with staying put. Not that changing domiciles was necessarily a bad idea. I just thought she should avoid doing something impulsive that she would regret later.

Minnie Sweet's history was replete with regrets. Any decision, and I mean ANY decision, was reviewed ad infinitum, with emphasis on the pros of the choice avoided, and endless repetition of the cons of the one selected. Conversations with Sidney went something like this:

"I can't get comfortable in the seats of this Buick, Sidney. I don't know why you had to sell the Oldsmobile."

"Don't start on that again, Minnie. Please! You know why I sold the Oldsmobile. You didn't like the way it idled. You said the vibrations annoyed you. You said that every time we stopped at a light you got nauseous. For seven years you said that. There was nothing wrong with the Olds and there's nothing wrong with the Buick."

"You don't have to shout at me, Sidney. I loved the Oldsmobile. I don't know where you got the idea I didn't like it. Anyway, we should have bought the Ford. That is some beautiful car. Sadie and Marv Holtz have the Ford. I've ridden in it. That's what we should have bought."

"Oy!" said Sidney and, wisely, he said nothing else.

Substitute this conversation for houses, vacations, restaurants, toasters, bathroom rugs, and purchases of all kinds, and you'll get the idea. So I knew what would happen. Minnie had made up her mind to move and wanted my approval. I had reached the point where I thought it might actually be a good idea.

She was slipping, visibly and rapidly. Always an impeccable housekeeper, her home was suddenly dirty. Things were growing in her refrigerator that weren't planted by farmers. She obviously wasn't eating well.

Plastic bags were stored in her oven, were forgotten, and would become a fire hazard if she ever decided to bake or broil. Thankfully, cooking wasn't one of her passions.

This had been a compulsively well-organized woman. Now, clutter was everywhere. Every flat surface in the house was covered with papers. Coffee tables, end tables, dining tables, kitchen counters, buffets, night tables, and chairs of all types.

Everything was papered with papers. And the papers were covered with dust. To pick up a sheet was to risk becoming enveloped in a cloud of six-month-old particles.

Some of the papers were important, like unpaid bills, insurance contracts, bank statements, and other things needing action. Some could be discarded, like ads, fundraising promotions, catalogues, and all sorts of junk mail. She was having a hard time telling the difference.

So maybe the house was getting to be too much for her. So maybe I should encourage her relocation. I called her to say so:

"Ma, this is Jerry."

"Hello sweetie, I love to hear your voice."

"Yeah. Listen Ma. I want to tell you something."

"I want to tell you something, too."

"Okay, you first."

"I have to sell the house."

"Okay, Ma. That's what I wanted to tell you. I'm in favor of that. What made you decide? It's just too big now, isn't it?"

"No. That's not it. I love this place."

"Then what?"

"It's Mr. Polsky across the street."

"Polsky? He seems like a nice man, what…?"

"That no-good! He yells at me when I back the car out of the driveway."

"He yells at you? Why?"

"He's a nasty, horrible stinker. That's why."

"Ma, did you back into his mailbox or something?"

Silence. Then:

"Absolutely not! He's just crazy and I don't want to live here anymore."

"You want to move because of Polsky?"

"I've listed the house."

"Already? You've already listed? With whom?"

"That nice Joe Kirby from the Lodge."

"Is he any good?"

"He told me he'd have the place sold in less than a month."

And that's how it went. Kirby never lifted a finger to sell the house. He was depending on the multi-list. He had priced it too high (to appease Minnie), and six months later nobody had even come to look. I made her change realtors. That "nice Joe Kirby" had let her down and was now known as the "gonif."

That's Yiddish for "swindler"…or worse.

PLAYING TO A PACKED HOUSE

It's hard to believe in 2005, but housing in many South Florida senior communities was overbuilt in the late 1980's, and prices in many sections had begun to decline. If you didn't live on the coast, chances were that your home was worth less in 1990 than in 1985.

Ring!

"Jerry, it's me."

"Hi Mom. What's up?"

"I have an offer, but I'm going to turn it down."

"Wait a minute. Don't do anything yet. The place has been on the market for a year and this is your first offer. What's wrong with it?"

"It's too little."

"What do you mean, too little?"

"Well, she'll give us our asking price, but..."

"Ma, that's terrific. Grab it!"

"Jerry, we put in a lot of extras. You know. The ceiling fans, the ceramic floor tiles, the..."

"You never get back what you spend on that sort of thing. Grab it! Who's the buyer?"

"Well, it's a little old widow. She's trying to steal the house. Anyway, I don't like her."

"Ma, you're a little old widow too. Maybe she doesn't like you either. Who cares? Sell the house."

"Your father and I loved this place. You know how handy he was. Look at all the improvements he made. Himself. With those talented hands. She wants to change it. I can't let that happen. What would he think?"

"Ma, he's gone, but I'll tell you what he'd think. He'd think you need to take the offer, that is unless you've changed your mind and want to stay in the house."

"I can't do that."

"Polsky?"

"Yes, Polsky, and stop making fun of me. The man is hateful."

"I'm not making fun of you. I just think you shouldn't have to move because of one man you don't like."

"It's not only him. It's the mice."

The mice again. I felt my heart sink when she said that. Every night she claimed to hear them scratching and squealing. Only there wasn't a single visible sign of infestation.

When I last visited Mom, I looked everywhere for droppings, for mouse holes, for anything that would corroborate her perception that her house was being overrun with the little rodents. When I said I couldn't find them, she said they were under the floorboards, especially in the bathroom. So I hired an exterminator to check it out. His conclusion: no mice!

Several months before her decision to sell her house, Minnie visited us up north. The first morning after she occupied our guest room, we found the closet stuffed and barricaded with her luggage, bedding, boxes, and anything that was within Mom's reach during the night.

On the other side of the back wall of this closet was another closet, this one in the bathroom off our master bedroom. It was a closet frequently visited by Nadine and me for shaving supplies, toiletries, and the like, especially before bedtime and in the morning.

A single sheet of wallboard that was anything but soundproof separated the two closets.

Here's the way the conversation went:

"Ma, what happened to your closet? Why is it crammed with all that junk?"

"Didn't you hear them? I was up all night."

"Hear who?"

"Not 'who.' 'What'?"

"What do you mean 'what'?"

"The mice, Jerry, the mice. Your house is full of them and they're all in that closet."

"Ma, we don't have any mice. I think you're hearing the noises that Nadine and I make moving things on the other side of your closet wall. Come, let me show you."

"You're making fun of me again, Jerry. I don't want to look in your closet. I don't have to. There are dozens of mice in my closet and I intend to keep them blocked in there."

And that's the way we left it. Now, months later, the mice seemed to have migrated to her house. Looking back, with what I now know, I believe this was a minor hallucination, an early sign of her developing dementia. At the time, I just got annoyed and exasperated.

Anyway, back to our telephone conversation about selling her house. For whatever reason, Polsky, mice, or some other whacky idea, Minnie had made up her mind to sell. Now she wanted my (and Sidney's) permission to do it. What could I do but grant it?

"Okay, okay," I said. "I think you should take the offer. Dad would agree."

"Do you really think so?"

"I know so. I asked him."

"I love you!"

"I love you too."

So the house was sold and the new owner wanted quick possession. For the seventh time in as many months I put my business on hold, tried to forget how much revenue I was forfeiting, and flew down to help find Minnie a new home. It wouldn't be the last of these trips.

We got lucky. In one weekend we found the perfect end unit condo in a pretty golf and tennis community. She wasn't going to play either sport, but the development was first class.

By now you can guess at the conversation, so I'll spare you the details. Minnie felt we paid too much and she didn't like the sellers.

Anyway, she purchased a lovely, 1200 square foot furnished condo, down from her 1800 square foot furnished house. It was a size I hoped she could manage. She had less than a month until moving day.

Minnie had always been a "squirrel," never throwing anything away, storing "whatever" for a rainy day that never arrived in a garage that could no longer accommodate a car.

When I looked at the clutter and examined the garage, I felt overwhelmed with what it was going to take to go through a lifetime of junk, sequester whatever was of real value and, somehow, persuade Minnie to toss the rest.

But, for now, I had a plane to catch. Thank God, I thought. Here's what I said:

"Ma, you have to start packing. I have to go home now, so can you manage this on your own?"

"I've packed all my life, remember? I'm an expert in packing."

"Okay. So I'll hire a mover and tell them that you'll do your own packing."

"Okay."

"Are you sure? I can have them pack for you, and save you the headache."

"Do they charge extra?"

"Of course."

"I'll pack myself.

"You can afford to have them pack."

"I'll pack myself."

"Also, Ma, don't get mad. You're going to a much smaller place. You have to throw away a lot of stuff in the garage. You have to clean up all the papers too; you know, pay the bills, file what I marked for filing, and dump the rest. Can you do that?"

"Do you take me for a dummy?"

"No, of course not. Listen, this is the most important part. You have to get rid of some furniture. It won't all fit."

"Okay."

"I'm serious, Ma. You really have to do this. I think you should sell the furniture in the new place, or give it to charity. That way you can keep your own furniture...the pieces that you've always loved. Will you make arrangements to do that, or should I?"

"I can do it, Jerry. You must really think I'm stupid or something."

"No Ma. I'm just trying to make it easier for you. And I'll come back on moving day to help. Okay?"

"I don't want you to take so much time off for me. I can manage by myself."

"I'm coming."

"I love you!"

"I love you too."

In subsequent weeks, the long distance phone conversations always included something like this:

"How's the packing going?"

"Okay."

"Have you started?"

"I got some boxes from Publix."

"But are you filling them?"

"I will. There's plenty of time."

"Why don't we have the movers pack for you?"

"I'll manage."

SQUEEZING 10 LBS OF POTATOES INTO A 5 LB SACK

As Minnie's moving day drew closer, I made my flight arrangements expecting that, when I arrived, I'd find a fully packed house ready to go onto the moving truck.

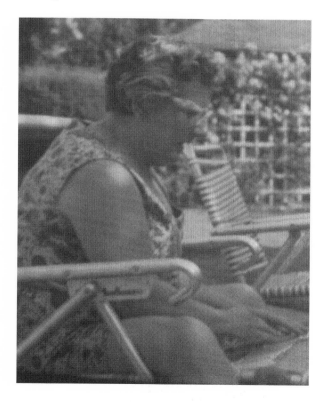

Truthfully, I did worry a bit that she might not have finished the job, but I dismissed that thought as unworthy and unthinkable. I was in for a surprise. Can you guess what it was?

If you guessed that she had gotten herself organized and had finished her packing, you would have been wide of the mark. Not only hadn't she finished packing, she had not even started.

Not a dish, teaspoon, garment, or trinket had moved one inch from where it had been on my last visit. Not a bill had been paid, nor a piece of paper disturbed. She hadn't done a thing.

That was the scene that greeted me when I arrived at her house in the late afternoon. The movers were scheduled to arrive the following morning. So what would you have done?

Here's what I did. I totally lost it. One should never yell at a parent, right? Well, one should never yell at anyone, really, but especially a parent...and especially a parent that was obviously having big problems coping with the routine activities of day-to-day living.

But denial is a powerful thing, and I had not yet admitted to myself the extent of Minnie's decline. To me, she was just being her old, obstinate, passive-aggressive self, digging in her heels and not doing what her son (formerly her husband and before that, her father) told her to do.

So I yelled. But she didn't get mad, defend herself, make excuses, explain her situation...nothing! In fact, she seemed bewildered by the whole thing.

So I took control. I called the movers late afternoon and was lucky enough to get the dispatcher who was getting the truck ready for the following morning. I described what I had found and asked him if it was too late to arrange for packers to come with the truck.

"No problem," he said.

"Phew!" I said. Then I downed a couple of aspirins and took Mom out to dinner. She was all smiley and relieved that I was taking charge. This was totally out of character for Minnie.

The move was supposed to have been a quick deal, only half a day. Now, with having to pack first, I knew that it would have to take a bit longer. Only I had no idea how much longer.

For starters, the truck arrived at 9 am, a half-hour late. For a moving van, that was really on time. After all, the crew was entitled to stop for a nice, leisurely breakfast on the way over, weren't they? And there were still almost three hours until their nice, leisurely lunch break would begin, so a lot could be accomplished in the morning. Right?

Wrong! We had originally been promised a crew of two men, the driver and an assistant. Since the dispatcher had said, "no problem," I assumed that we would get at least four. Two to pack and two to load the truck. You know the old adage about "assume making an ass out of you and me (ass-u-me)?" He-Haw!

All we got were the same two guys who were originally scheduled. They had their arms twisted until they agreed to do both the packing AND the move. If they had known what faced them they would have run like hell.

So K'wami and José walked in, said hello, looked around, and turned white, which was a pretty good trick for two gentlemen of color. That was only the first of their shocks that day. "Did the dispatcher tell you I called?" I asked.

"Yup," said K'wami. He was the older of the two, the driver, and the guy in charge. He would also turn out to be a man of few words and most of these words would be justified complaints about what the dispatcher had gotten him into.

"Then you know that everything has to be packed first."

"Yup."

"So where are the packers?"

"You're looking at them."

"You're gonna need more help. It will take two men forever."

"It's Saturday. Me and José is all they got. Lucky for you we was scheduled. From what I see, not so lucky for us."

I remembered that we had agreed to pay extra for a Saturday move so it could happen with me present. Of course they would be short staffed on the weekend.

"I'll help," I said. We were paying by the hour so I was motivated. Minnie was nowhere to be seen. She had started to yell at our guests the minute they arrived, and I took her aside and begged her to back off. Since then I could hear her in her bedroom. I could hear drawers were opening and closing, but I didn't know what was going on.

"What should we do with all these papers?" asked K'wami. "I can't pack the furniture it's sitting on until it's removed, and I don't want the responsibility of touching the stuff."

"I don't blame you. Give me some cartons and I'll take care of the papers," I said, feeling overwhelmed. "Meanwhile, get started with the kitchenware."

While K'wami was getting the cartons, I checked the noises in the bedroom. Mom and José were in mortal combat over the contents of her dresser drawers. The piece must have weighed 1000 pounds.

He wanted to remove the drawers to make the dresser lighter and easier to handle. Mom wanted him to move the dresser onto the truck without removing the drawers. Why? Beats me, but José was ready to quit and the day was just getting started.

This discussion was interrupted by a groan coming from the garage. Thinking that K'wami had hurt himself on some of Sidney's tools, I rushed to his aid. The groan was due to psychic pain, not physical distress.

"What's wrong, K'wami?" I asked, as if I didn't know. At Minnie's request, Dad had installed wall to wall tiered shelving throughout the garage and every inch of it was crammed with dust covered boxes, most of which contained nothing worth saving and, certainly, not worth paying to move. Besides, the new condo had no garage, just a small storage closet.

With Minnie out of earshot, I quickly sampled most of the shelves and granted K'wami permission to leave it behind. My plan was to examine the stuff myself and dump most of it. I didn't know how Minnie would react to this plan but, at the moment, I really didn't care.

And that's the way the morning went. By Noon, Minnie had quieted down and things were getting organized. It was clear, however, that this move was going to last late into the night and would cost a fortune.

And the movers hadn't even discovered the worst yet. That would come at around 3 PM when K'wami and José made the first trip with the truck to the new condo, while I continued to pack unbreakables myself (for insurance reasons, I had to let the crew pack anything fragile).

"Did you know that the new place is furnished," asked K'wami when he and José returned. He sounded disgusted.

Of course. I had forgotten. I had asked Mom to get rid of that stuff. Another ball seems to have dropped. "I know." I said.

"It's also much smaller than this house."

"I know."

"What furniture are you leaving behind here?"

"Ma," I called and, as she emerged from her bedroom where she had been resting, I asked, "What furniture are you leaving behind?"

"What do you mean, 'leaving behind'?"

"Everything won't fit, Ma. You were supposed to get rid of the stuff that came with the new place."

"I decided I like it."

"Okay. That's fine. But then there's no room for all your old furniture."

"I'll make it fit."

"Mrs. Sweet," said K'wami, sounding more courteous and patient than I would have been, "the new place is too small. You won't have room to walk. You'll have floor to ceiling boxes in every room. Furniture pieces will get stacked on top of each other."

"Jerry, tell him I want it all moved."

"You heard her, K'wami. You've warned her, so you're not responsible. It all goes."

So, shaking his head, and muttering under his breath, K'wami called for José and, by 9 PM, the move from Hell was finished. Minnie, of course, was mad at them and didn't want me to tip them. When she wasn't looking, I gave them double the usual amount. They deserved more.

K'wami's predictions of apartment congestion turned out to have been optimistic. But, again, (thank God) I had a plane to catch the next day.

"Ma," I said. "How can I leave you like this? You don't have an inch of space to maneuver. I don't know how you'll even unpack."

"I'll manage," she said.

"We could pay to have them unpack you," I said, wondering even as I did, how this would work. I had no doubt that K'wami and José were history. Nothing could persuade them to come back.

"Should we do that?" I continued.

"I love you," she said, shaking her head.

"I love you too."

Somehow Minnie did manage. I don't know how she did it but, gradually, whenever I visited her in her new condo, I noticed that there were fewer boxes and more space.

I suspected that she had found someone to help her. She could be very persuasive playing the "Damsel in Distress" role, and there was always an aging knight nearby willing to come to her aid.

"Ma," I said on one of my visits, "the place is beginning to shape up. I don't know how you've done it, but I'm impressed. Have you had help?"

Her silent reply was a mischievous smile, so I continued, "Where did you put all that stuff?"

"It's in the storage room," she said, still smiling.

"But Ma, there isn't that much space in the storage room. Did you give a lot of it away?"

"I didn't have to. I told you I'd manage, didn't I? You didn't have any confidence in me."

"Of course I did. You did me proud. I feel so much better about your new place now that it's begun to look so homey. Listen, can I take a look at the storage area?"

Her smile went away. "Why?"

"Listen, Ma. Don't you think I should know where things are? What if something happens? What if you're, God forbid, in the hospital and you ask me to bring you something from storage?"

A big sigh and a reluctant, "Okay, let me get the keys."

The keys? Why plural? The rules say that each resident is only permitted to have one locked storage area. Somehow, Minnie had finagled a couple of widower neighbors into letting her "borrow" their storage spaces.

Since neither of the men were "collectors," their storage areas were empty and they were happy to oblige. As I say, Mom's expertise lay in helping others to feel good about helping her.

So she had three adjacent storage cages, jammed side to side and top to bottom with many of the unopened boxes and some of the furnishings that previously crammed her apartment.

There was no way anyone could know where anything was within these cages, nor could anything have been easily retrieved even if it's location could be identified. Yup, Minnie had managed all right.

I returned her keys without comment. She silently accepted them back with a smile.

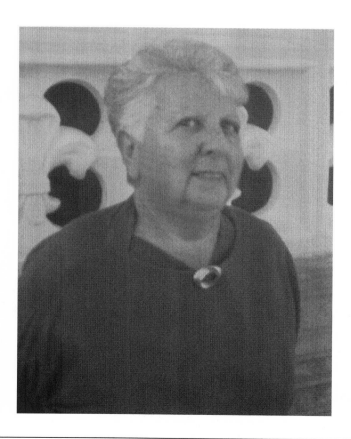

TRUTH AND CONSEQUENCES

"How do you like my ceramic floor tiles?" Minnie asked during one of my visits soon after her move to her new condo.

"They're very nice. Are they new?" I asked, not remembering what the place came with.

"Brand new. So is the ceiling fan in the dining area, the lighting in the kitchen, and the sun proof coating on the windows in the enclosed porch."

She knew what I would think. I was being led into a fight. I was expected to challenge her decision to spend the money to do these improvements. I knew it was money down the tubes. Money that she might need to live on someday.

It was one more example of a growing list of poor judgments she was making; judgments that could come back to hurt her in the future. But what could I say? There were bigger issues on my mind that day, and I didn't need a knock down, dragged out argument.

"I'm happy you're happy," was all I said.

Minnie looked sad at having been deprived of her psychic exercise. She loved a good fight. However, I had a mission on this trip and I could not risk being distracted from achieving it.

As an only son living far away from an isolated and elderly parent, it was clear that I would have to play an increasing role in the care of my mother. The problem was that I was a long distance caregiver.

As she became more and more needy, something that was inevitable with her advancing age, how would I know when to drop everything and come running? I had a business to run and had to choose my timing very carefully.

Things that sounded like a crisis on the telephone often turned out to be relatively minor and were virtually resolved by the time I could get away and fly down. On the other hand, things that sounded fairly minor often escalated into full fledged crises, with me still "up north" trying to quarterback things by phone.

Who could I rely on for good advice as to whether I was really needed? Her sister, my Aunt Charlotte, was there part of the year and was a great comfort. But even she wasn't always available. Nor was it fair to expect her to be. So, who to turn to?

Remember, Minnie never had the same doctor for more than a couple of months before she alienated him and his office staff, or vice versa. So there wasn't a medical professional that I could call about her. Every so often, at my request, she would provide the name and phone number of her current physician and claim that she appreciated my interest and help.

Somehow, however, by the time I got around to calling the latest doctor, Minnie would no longer be a patient. Coincidence? Or did she want to keep her health issues private. If so, I could respect that. But she was increasingly forgetful and rebellious about following medical advice.

When she didn't like the advice, you know what she did. Right! She changed doctors. She was also pharmaceutically non-compliant. Every medication prescribed for her blood pressure, anxiety attacks, breathing problems, whatever, seemed to cause such bad side effects that she felt she had to stop taking them. Or she just plain forgot. Either way, she was not getting any benefit from them and her health was getting noticeably worse.

I had a plan to help me stay better informed about Minnie's daily needs, but it would require her willing cooperation. A new profession had recently emerged to help relatives of elderly family members supervise and coordinate care and services for their loved ones. Its practitioners were known as Geriatric Care Managers and I wanted to hire one for Mom.

A national association of these GCM's had formed for the purpose of promoting professionalism among its membership. It provided contact information for those of their members that practiced in South Florida. In fact, I had already spoken to several local GCM's, had selected one, and was ready to go. But would Mom buy into this idea? I had my doubts.

There were all sorts of services that these professionals said they could provide to Minnie, depending upon their individual backgrounds and training. These included, among other things, clinical services, transportation, shopping assistance, emotional support, financial management, liaison with social services, or just plain old companionship.

Perhaps the most attractive feature of this service was the potential of having an objective, third party, on the scene, able to monitor the situation and to report regularly to me about Minnie's needs.

It was like buying a surrogate care-giving relative, I thought, to be there for Mom when I could not. Without question, there would be some tough choices to be made down the road, some of which might be heart wrenching and guilt producing. Like the possibility of having to arrange for nursing home care, for example.

I didn't want to face such decisions alone, always to wonder whether I had done the right thing for Minnie. Here was a way, I thought, to have a partner to assist me to evaluate each situation, and to advise me on the best professional options for my mother. It was the perfect setting, I thought, for a Geriatric Care Manager.

"Ma," I said. "Let's talk."

"What do you think we've been doing?'

"No, I mean about something important."

"Oh, so you think my getting settled in my new place isn't important?"

"You know that's not what I mean. Listen, Ma, I'm worried about you when I'm not here. You're refrigerator's almost empty and, frankly Ma, don't get upset, but some of the stuff you have in there is inedible. Are you eating right?"

"Do I look undernourished?"

She had a point. If anything, she had put on weight. But that didn't mean she was getting proper nourishment.

"You look great," I lied, "but I want you to stay that way. You know, while I'm here, I could arrange for 'Meals On Wheels' to deliver your dinner a couple of times each week."

"What are you talking about? I used to volunteer for 'Meals On Wheels.' The people Dad and

I delivered food to were old and decrepit. I don't need that service."

"Ma, that was ten years ago. You're ten years older and alone now…"

"I don't need that service."

"But…"

"Listen, Jerry. Speaking of eating right, let's go grab a bite. I'm hungry."

"Ma, we just had lunch half an hour ago."

"I didn't have anything."

"Yes you did. You had a tuna fish sandwich, half a grapefruit and a big piece of Danish."

"That was yesterday."

"It was half an hour ago."

"No it wasn't. Why do you make up these stories? Let's go eat."

"We just ate. I'm not hungry yet."

And so the argument raged with Mom getting more furious by the minute. When it finally dawned on me that she wasn't being difficult, but really couldn't remember eating lunch, I surrendered and took her to the neighborhood deli. Incredibly, she downed a huge corned beef sandwich while I nursed a cup of coffee and looked around the deli.

Walkers and canes were everywhere. A thin, frail looking woman about Minnie's age, bent with osteoporosis, was laboriously making her way past our table with a walker.

"Look at her," Minnie said, too loudly and with a tone of disgust in her voice, "why do they let them in here? This place is getting to be like a nursing home."

Embarrassed because the woman had to have heard, I waited until she was out of earshot, and I said, "Ma, she heard you. That wasn't very nice."

"She didn't hear a thing. She has double hearing aids."

"Which probably enabled her to hear exactly what you said. I think you wanted her to hear you. That was cruel."

"I don't care. They shouldn't let people like that in here."

I didn't argue. This was becoming a constant. Minnie had less and less compassion and empathy for elderly people who showed outward signs of deterioration.

The more I defended them and criticized her for her rudeness, the louder she would argue her case that people needing walkers, wheelchairs and canes should be confined to institutions, or at least kept out of public places. Her disparaging comments mortified and disappointed me.

I remembered a kind and considerate mother. Where had she gone?

Years later I would recall these episodes and recognize them for what they were—her fear that she was next. Rejecting handicapped people was, for her, like rejecting the handicaps themselves. But, at the time, all I felt was anger. I wasn't sure about what was happening to Minnie, but I knew she needed help.

Back at the condo, I tried again. "Ma, I want you to do something for me."

"For you, sweetie, anything,"

"Look, I know you don't think you need any help, but I need to have peace of mind about you. I have a suggestion about how to accomplish this."

Since she seemed receptive, I explained about the Geriatric Care Manager and why I wanted her to have such a service.

"It's for me, Ma. Give it a try."

"How much does it cost?"

"It's a community service," I lied, "so there is no charge." Actually, I would pay for it, and it wasn't cheap, but I'd been advised not to tell this to Mom.

Experience had taught the GCM I was talking with that elderly parents tend to resist accepting the service if they think their kids are paying for it. And they certainly would never agree to pay for it themselves.

"Honey, if it will give you peace of mind, I'm agreeable. I don't need it, but I'll try it for you. Now, I want you to do something for me."

Uh, oh! "Sure, Ma. What is it?"

"Promise me that you'll never put me in a nursing home."

Sometimes a lie is a blessing. I've already admitted to telling several falsehoods that I thought were in Minnie's best interests, so why on Earth I suddenly felt a need to be totally honest I'll never know. But I did.

Here's how I (stupidly, in retrospect) answered her request for my promise:

"No."

"No? What do you mean 'no'?" Her voice was rising and her face was flushed. I could literally see her blood pressure going up. Why couldn't I recognize her terror?

"Ma, how can I promise? First of all, I would never 'put' you anywhere. But who knows what the future might bring? How do we know you'd never need a nursing home? Of course, I'll do everything in my power to help you avoid it, but what if your condition at the time requires it?"

"Promise me!"

"Ma, I'd be lying if I did. I'll try, but…"

"You mean you won't promise?"

"Not 'won't,' can't. What if you're in the hospital or something, and…"

I didn't finish the sentence. She was absolutely hysterical. I don't recall her exact words, but my mother had never before said such abusive things to me. It was a shocking first, soon to become a regular feature of our relationship.

ALTERNATIVE LONG DISTANCE SERVICE

Flo Golden charged $25 an hour for her Geriatric Care Management service and, at first, I was happy to pay it. She came highly recommended, was a member of the GCM professional association, and she lived near Minnie. She sounded personable and intelligent on the phone. What more could I ask?

Surprisingly, Minnie continued to sound receptive to such assistance, and so I set up her first appointment with Flo. I then waited with the proverbial "baited breath," certain that Minnie would find a way to sabotage the scheme.

If she did, it wouldn't be the first time that she used overt cooperation as a mask for killing a venture. Was she really okay with this? As much as I pondered it, I could not predict the outcome.

Flo did an initial assessment interview and provided a written report that recommended engaging her for ongoing guidance and assistance to Minnie. She felt that Mom needed someone nearby to confide in, to analyze why she alienated others, and to prevent situations like the Polsky wars from happening again with her new neighbors.

She also said that Minnie had definite symptoms of early dementia. The import of this news registered with me, but I had no idea yet of its long-term implications for Minnie's life...and for mine.

Based on my conversations with Flo, I was led to expect at least the following services:

- Management of personal affairs, including referrals to financial, legal and/or medical professionals, as necessary.

- Care-planning assessments.

- Coordination of in-home services, if and when needed.

- Crisis intervention.

- Counseling and support.

- Weekly communication with me.

This last was, from my point of view, the most important single benefit of the service I thought I was buying. And for the first month or so, Flo did stay in touch, maybe not weekly, but often enough so that I had a sense of what was happening with Minnie.

In all fairness to Flo, I believe she had every intention of providing all of the benefits she promised...and I think she may even have tried. But she was no match for Minnie, and it didn't take long for Flo to lose control.

Here's what Minnie had to say to me via long distance telephone:

"What a nice person, Jerry. This Flo, I mean. I really like her."

"Great, Ma. Remember, her job is to stay in touch with you and to keep me informed about your needs."

"I don't really need anything."

"I know. This is for my peace of mind, remember?"

"I know you worry. So, I'll keep seeing Flo. I'll do it for you. Anyway, she took me to lunch and we had a great talk."

"Really? She took you to lunch?" I didn't recall that being part of the deal. Who paid for lunch, I wondered? And would I be billed $25 an hour for the time Flo spent at lunch with Minnie? Of course I would. Hmmm?

"Not only that. She took me to my doctor appointment too."

Chauffer services? Another thing that hadn't been discussed. Minnie was still driving, so why was this necessary?

"No kidding. How did that happen?"
"I asked her to. I didn't feel like driving. Wasn't that nice of her?"

"Oh yes. Very nice. Let me ask. Did she wait in the waiting room while you were with the doctor?"

"You bet. She had to take me home afterwards, so she waited for me. I really like her."

So, it seemed as though I was paying Flo an hourly fee for the time she spent having lunches with Minnie (plus the cost of the lunches which were listed as "Related Expenses" on Flo's bills), for chauffer services, and for waiting around in doctors' offices.

I thought I had hired a GCM. Instead, I appeared to have "bought" a new best friend for a woman who had alienated all of her "free" friends. And I couldn't complain to Minnie since she thought Flo's services were free. So I called Flo hoping to hear a good explanation for what was happening.

"Flo," I said. "I haven't heard from you directly in months. I thought weekly reports were part of your service."

"Yes...well...there really wasn't anything significant to report."

"But you're seeing Mom a lot, in fact more hours per week than we had agreed to, and you're billing me for the extra time. If there's nothing significant to report, why is this necessary?"

"Your mother is very lonely, Jerry, and her self-esteem is low. She needs a regular visit from a friend, and I'm all she has in Florida at the moment."

"I don't understand. In the past twenty years, she established three Hadassah Chapters and served as President of each of them. She was Chair of a chapter of B'nai Brith Women. She was active with the Jewish war Veterans, and a Matron of the Eastern Star. She was Director of Volunteers for her city, and a member of its Library Board. And much, much more. But you know all this. Where are the dozens and dozens of friends she and Sidney made in all these groups? Mom has been a human dynamo. How can you be all she has?"

"I don't know what happened to her friends, but they're not around. She says they only care about themselves. She's very depressed."

"Okay, that sounds like an acceptable basis for your involvement, but I still don't know why you're not communicating with me directly. Also, how are you diagnosing Mom's loneliness and self-esteem...her depression?"

"She told me herself. I listen to what she says. You should too."

Whoa! That sounded kind of judgmental, but I ignored it for the moment.

"She told you? Is that sufficient? Don't you have some sort of professional tool for these kinds of things?"

"Listen, Jerry, Minnie is very needy," Flo said, sidestepping my question. "What am I supposed to do when she calls me every day and begs me to take her to lunch or to the doctor?"

"Well, since I'm the one who pays you, Flo, I'd expect you to call me in advance to authorize the extra time. Minnie can be very manipulative..."

"You're telling me!"

"Exactly. So, from now on, I expect you to say 'no' when Mom asks for more time than we've contracted for. If she wants to know why, tell her it's my wish."

"I don't recommend that. You know, Jerry, she's very angry at you. One of the main things she wants to do at lunch is complain about you and Nadine."

Uh oh! Minnie's sister Charlotte and one of my own children had been reporting frequent phone calls with venomous attacks upon me. They seem to have started shortly after Flo's services began.

"What exactly does she say about us, Flo?"

"That's just it. She's very vague about it. Something about nursing homes, I think. I'm trying to get her to open up about it. It's important that she learn how to express these hostile feelings."

What was going on here, I wondered? I had needed an objective ally to help me plan for Minnie's needs but, suddenly, there were hostile feelings that needed expressing, and two adversarial camps: Minnie and Flo versus me and Nadine.

The GCM concept made sense to me, but perhaps I selected the wrong person. She was adding to my stress, rather than relieving it…not at all what I had in mind by hiring her.

Maybe it was time to cancel Flo. It would be hard to explain to Minnie who, clearly, had co-opted this so-called professional's judgment and behavior. However, the emotional and financial costs were becoming burdensome. I made a snap decision.

"Flo, I want you to stop seeing her."

"What do you mean?"

"I'm not happy with your services. I'm sorry to have to say that, but there it is."

After a time, and softly, "Your mother needs me, Jerry. She won't be pleased about this. What if I continue to see her anyway?"

"No problem, but if you do, then you can send your bill to her." I was beginning to understand where all the so-called "hostile feelings" might be coming from. Minnie was not the only manipulative talent on the block.

"What do you mean?"

"I mean I won't pay you anymore."

"But Minnie can't pay me. She doesn't know I charge for my time. She just thinks I'm a friend. It would ruin our relationship if I billed her. You're the one who hired me."

"Exactly. And now I'm firing you."

Actually, Minnie took the news all right. I had to confess to her that Flo's time wasn't free. That did it. She said she was totally supportive of dropping Flo and she took delight in reminding me that she only got involved with Flo to please me.

However, it turned out to be much easier to start up with Flo than it was to end it. Several months after I terminated her service, a bill arrived for two hours of her time, along with a brief written report.

She stated that Minnie had sounded distressed on the phone, but she did not say who initiated the call. She reported taking Minnie to lunch again because she felt my mother needed a sympathetic listener

"Flo," I said, when I called her, "I'm not going to pay your bill. I thought I had made my position clear."

"But you mother asked me to meet her. She was so lonely, Jerry. She is very vulnerable and she really needs me."

I was beginning to wonder who was needier, Minnie or Flo. "That may be true, Flo, but why didn't you just call me first, as I had asked, to tell me you were getting involved again?"

"You're right. I should have done that. It won't happen again."

"Right. It won't. I'm not paying your bill."

That seemed to do it. Neither Minnie nor I ever heard from Flo again. I still felt I needed a local ally, though, and so I did what I probably should have done in the first place. I contacted a Jewish agency in Minnie's community and learned about its reasonably priced geriatric evaluation and support service.

Shortly thereafter, a real geriatric professional, one of its social workers, Gloria Gelman, was on Minnie's case, evaluating Mom's needs, conducting herself professionally, and reporting regularly to me.

Gloria's service was everything I had hoped for in hiring Flo, and didn't get. She soon discovered that Minnie had known all along that Flo was charging me, and that my mother was deliberately running up the clock as her way of killing the arrangement. At least, that's what she told Gloria.

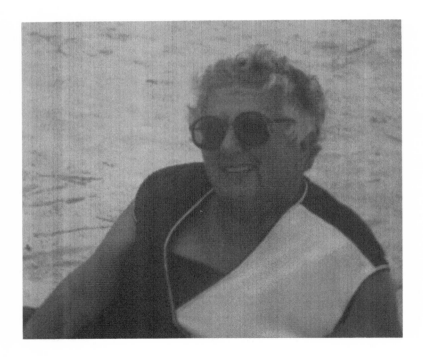

It didn't take long for Gloria to figure out that Minnie had some real emotional and cognitive problems, that she was probably at the beginning stage of some sort of dementia, and that the symptoms were certain to get worse.

She began to prepare me and Minnie for a day, in the not too distant future, when my mother would need to move again, this time into a more sheltered environment.

But that's a story for another chapter.

BOOMERANG BUBBE

"Jerry, I've made a big decision." Minnie's voice on the phone was rational and firm.

For most of Minnie's life, she became overwrought when faced with a decision, even a little one like choosing a dinner from a restaurant menu. She was the living embodiment of that old joke. You know the one.

QUESTION: Do you have trouble making decisions?

ANSWER: Well...yes and no!

She would go back and forth, back and forth, making a choice, regretting it, changing her mind, regretting it, over and over and over. Sometimes weeks, and even months would go by, during which Minnie would whine and complain about how she should have made a different choice.

She was never satisfied that, whatever her decision, it was the best one under the circumstances. There was always a better option out there that she thought she should have chosen.

So, her announcement about having made a BIG decision unsettled me. What was she up to now?

"Great, Ma," I said, finally, with a tightening in the pit of my stomach. "What is it?"

"I've decided to come north to live near you and Nadine."

Mixed feelings! This was just what I wanted and I had been lobbying Minnie hard for it lately. I never really expected it to happen. You know the old adage about being careful what you wish for...?

"Terrific, Ma. I didn't think you were ready to move again."

"I didn't think so either, but Gloria convinced me. I'm not getting any younger, Jerry. My place is with my children."

Gloria! God bless her! This was exactly the kind of decision I could not make alone. When making such enormous changes in the life of an elderly parent, especially one with dementia, how can a caregiver know the right thing to do? Some had siblings to help with the process. I did not...and I was too close to it, too emotionally involved.

Gloria Gelman, social worker, was my counselor as well as Minnie's, and her advice was to get Mom to move near me as soon as possible. Gloria had been calling me regularly about Minnie's condition, and was reporting major slippage.

Until now, Minnie had dug in her heels. She was not moving again, and certainly not moving north. I don't know how Gloria sold it, but Minnie had done a complete reversal. For the most part, I was pleased. Frightened, but pleased.

"This is great news, Ma. When do you want to do this?"

"As soon as you can get me into those senior apartments we saw the last time I visited you."

These apartments are a community-based project with modern facilities located on two suburban campuses. Each building offers somewhat different programs to its elderly clientele, depending upon the needs of each individual.

Some units offer totally independent housing, some provide a partial support environment, and some supply complete assisted living services. Each campus also boasts a large community center with swimming pools, gyms, and lots of special programs for seniors.

In the building we were considering for Minnie, there is a social work staff and an activities director. It would be hard, I thought, for Minnie to avoid getting involved in the building's active social life. She would no longer be as isolated as she seemed to be in her Florida condo.

Also, she would be well nourished for a change, since her rent would include five dinners per week in a communal dining room that would supplement the limited cooking facilities in her apartment. For all these reasons, I felt good about bringing Minnie up to live in such an environment.

There was just one negative, but it was a big one. There were large waiting lists for all but the studio apartments, and the latter were understandably unpopular because of their diminutive size.

If Minnie was willing to take a studio, she could move up any time she wanted. If not, there was at least a one-year wait.

So I said, "Ma, there's a long waiting list for the one bedrooms, but you can probably get into a studio right away."

"I don't want to wait. My place is with my children."

"I think so too, but I want you to realize that the studio apartments are single room affairs with a small kitchen alcove and a bathroom. One side of the room has a bed and the other is the living area. Very compact."

"I'll manage."

"Seriously, Ma. It could be very uncomfortable for a while. You'd have priority for a one bedroom that opened, but that could take a year or so. In the meantime, you'd have less space than you've ever lived in before. I don't want you to regret the move, or to be unhappy about your new apartment. Maybe we should wait."

"No! My place is with my children. Get me a studio. I want to come north."

"Are you sure? I don't want you getting mad at me if you don't like it. I want it to be your decision. I'll tell you what. Come for a visit, interview the admissions director, see the apartment, and decide for yourself."

So that's what she did. She came, she looked, and she said, "It is small, but I don't care. My place is with my children. Move me up."

"Do you want help finding a moving company? You didn't like the last one."

"No, I know a nice man here who manages a different one. I'll use him."

"What about putting your condo on the market? I can help with the realtor."

"I'm not going to sell it yet."

Uh oh! Red flag! That sounded like an "insurance policy" scheme to me, a back up plan just in case she decided to move back.

Even Minnie wouldn't go to all the trouble of moving her household fifteen hundred miles, only to scamper back to Florida the first time that the adjustment proved difficult...or would she? Better not take the chance. This was Minnie we were dealing with. Anything was possible.

"Ma, you have to sell it."

"Why do I have to?"

"If you are moving up here permanently, why would you need to keep it?"

Silence. Then, "I know a realtor. He's that nice man that helped Sonia Blatt. I'll call him."

"Ma, don't play games. Nadine and I really want you here, but..."

"You mean it? You want me there?"

"Of course we do, but..."

"I love you."

"I love you too, but let me finish. We want you here, but only if you are willing to make a permanent commitment. Keeping your condo is a signal that you're not really ready to do that."

"I'm ready."

"Are you sure?"

"I'm sure. I'll sell the condo."

She really did list it with the realtor and, after a time, I trusted her and stopped asking. Preparations were made for the move, with packing arrangements contracted far in advance this time. I visited once or twice to help her get organized. She agreed to my suggestion to sell the condo furnished and to bring a minimum amount of stuff with her.

If moving from her house to her condo was like stuffing ten pounds of potatoes into a five-pound sack, this move into a studio apartment would be like putting the remaining five pounds into a one-pound sack.

I didn't even want to think about it...but I should have. She played me beautifully. First of all, contrary to our agreement about selling the condo furnished, she left not a stitch of anything behind. Secondly, it was only after she arrived that I discovered she fired the realtor, and she didn't want to hire a replacement.

Minnie continued to deny that her intent was to hang onto the condo "just in case," and I wanted to believe her. But there were other issues distracting me.

The moving truck, for example, arrived at the apartments one day after I retrieved Minnie from the airport and installed her in her third floor studio. There was one very slow elevator serving the floor.

I worried about how the movers were going to get her things up to her apartment expeditiously. If I knew the actual size of the load that was coming, my concern would have turned to panic. We were paying by the hour again. Don't ask. It's how that "nice man" Minnie had talked about set things up.

Anyway, it turned out that I was way off base. I had been worried about the wrong things. The delivery did not take the movers long at all. They carried the heavy furniture up, but her boxes, her dozens of boxes, they left downstairs, outside on the sidewalk. That was their policy at apartment houses with small, slow elevators, they explained.

"You can't just leave it there," I protested. "I'm the only one that can finish the move. It will take me forever. Some of that stuff is very heavy. What if it rains? Things will get ruined."

"Sorry," said the driver. "I have another delivery to do today. I'll never make it if I have to move all those cartons up on that elevator. I gotta go now. By the way, here's the bill. I need a certified check or cash."

I gasped. Even with their abbreviated effort on delivery, the bill from the moving company was enormous. After all, it was an interstate move and it took a huge chunk out of the money that Sidney left Minnie. For some reason, that seemed not to concern her as much as it did me.

The building staff was also not available to help carry boxes. That was their policy too, they explained. Their worker's compensation insurance policy wouldn't cover any injuries sustained from such activities.

So Charles "Jerry" Atlas had his work cut out for him. After many hours of shlepping and hauling, with the aid of a small hand truck I brought from our basement, I got all the boxes moved. I ached all over but, inexplicably, my back had not gone out.

You should have seen that studio. In a classic case of deja vue, every inch of space from wall to wall and floor to ceiling was crammed with cartons.

Somehow I was able to make a narrow passage between boxes from the bed to the bathroom, and to the front door. That pathway was the only space not jammed with things.

If you get the idea that Minnie brought virtually everything she owned with her again, you are correct.

Fortunately, she agreed to send much of her living and dining room furniture to her grandchildren.

Whether they wanted it or not, they were polite and accepted the stuff, but who knows? But that still left her whole bedroom set and an assortment of odd pieces to try to squeeze into the studio.

I didn't know if Minnie could adjust to such conditions and it wasn't long after she moved in that she started to blame me for "putting" her into such unsatisfactory housing.

She conveniently forgot my gentle efforts to persuade her not to take the studio, as well as her own preview and endorsement of the apartment. It was completely her decision, but what difference did that make now?

The tight, cramped, crowded studio apartment was unlivable, she said. According to Minnie, the food was inedible, and the climate was drying out her skin.

Also, as usual, she didn't like the people, which probably meant that she said some impolite things and was then rejected by the recipients of her comments. It was the same pattern that Gloria Gelman and Flo Golden described about Minnie's lost friendships in Florida.

She had been such a great social animal, with tons and tons of friends, that it was hard for me to grasp the fact that her "new" personality drove people away from her. But that's the way it was and, from Minnie's perspective, all the horrid things that happened to her up north were totally my fault.

Minnie Sweet moved up north to be with "her children" on St. Patrick's Day. By Memorial Day, exactly ten weeks later, she and all of her possessions were enroute back to her Florida condo along with another big bill from the moving company.

One postscript to this chapter. When Minnie arrived at the apartments she gave me Sidney's Bonneville as a birthday present. It was with a big fanfare that she announced her intention to give up driving forever. By this time the Bonneville was no longer new, and all the scars of Minnie's tenure with it were visible on its dented and scratched body.

I really didn't want the car. I didn't need it and, if I did, I would have chosen something new. Still, it was a low mileage vehicle, and the best part was that Minnie would not be driving. I would no longer have to worry about her killing herself or someone else while behind the wheel. So I graciously accepted the gifted vehicle.

When Minnie announced her intent to return to Florida, I knew she would soon realize that she no longer had the wheels she'd come to depend on in her past life. She would have a tough time surviving in her old neighborhood without the Bonneville, but I didn't think it wise or safe for her to drive again.

What happened next is the amazing subject of the following chapter.

SHOULD A CAREGIVER BE A CARGIVER?

Nadine grabbed the phone. "It's your Mom," she said.

"Again?" I groaned. "It's the fifth call in less than an hour."

"Be patient, Jerry," said my wife, her hand over the mouthpiece. "Moving day is Thursday. You have to expect her to be somewhat anxious."

"I suppose. Okay, give me the phone."

Resigned to expect the unexpected, I accepted the receiver with foreboding.

My mouth felt dry as I said, for the fifth time that morning, "Hi, Mom."

"Jerry, I just realized something. This is important. How will I get around when I'm back in Florida?"

I had been expecting this. Hoping it wouldn't happen, but expecting it all the same. Knowing full well what she meant, I asked her anyway. "What do you mean, 'get around'?"

"I mean, I will have to drive."

"It's not safe, Ma. You were driving the wrong way on one-way streets before you came up here in March. The Bonneville has more dents than a golf ball. You don't have to drive. There are shuttle services for seniors in Florida. Also, retired guys offering cheap cab rides are a dime a dozen."

"Jerry, I want my car back."

There it was. The moment I had been dreading, but which was as inevitable as the sun rising.

In the September 2003 issue of the AARP Bulletin, John Eberhard, former senior research psychologist at the National Highway Traffic Safety Administration, wrote, "Telling seniors they can no longer drive is as hard as telling them they have terminal cancer."

I knew exactly what he meant. This was my mother speaking. The woman who birthed me, almost losing her life in the process.

The Mom who diapered, fed, nursed, and loved me through all the ups and downs of childhood and (poor lady) my adolescence. How do I defy her? Yet I had no doubt that she, and the world around her, would not be well served by her driving.

In fact, I couldn't return the Bonneville even if I wanted to. Anticipating this very moment, I sold the car at a throwaway price. I planned to put the proceeds into Minnie's bank account when I could do so without alerting her prematurely as to the source of the funds.

Why did I sell the car? So I wouldn't be tempted to give it back to her when she demanded it. It turned out to have been a smart move. Painful, but smart.

Now, all I could do was say, "Ma, you can't have the Bonneville back," and wait for the explosion. It wasn't long in coming. To protect her dignity, I won't quote the things she said to me during the temper tantrum that followed.

I pointed out that the Bonneville was my birthday gift and that she shouldn't be asking for it back. No effect.

I told her that I was forced to trade the car because it was falling apart mechanically. She didn't believe me.

I told her that I really no longer had the Bonneville to give. That, at least, was totally true, but she didn't believe that either.

After what seemed like hours of her protests and pleas, but was actually only about fifteen minutes, my heart was breaking, but my resolve was still solid. She asked again, a bit more calmly now, "So, will you give me back my car or not?"

I got as far as, "Ma, I love you but I can't. I really don't have it any...Hello?"

There was nobody at the other end of the line. It was my toughest moment in a lifetime of tough moments as Minnie Sweet's beloved son.

Minnie never referred to this conversation again and never again asked for her car. In fact, she became almost excessively cooperative during the rest of the few days prior to her leaving.

She was scheming something. Of that I was certain, and I knew that sooner or later I would find out exactly what it was.

It had been emotionally challenging for me to have her come to live near me in the first place, but I felt it was important for both of us to be together during the latter part of her life. Now, her impulsive return to her Florida condo left me feeling angry and judgmental.

The cost of these frequent long distance moves were depleting the dollars that she'd need in her later years for food and housing, but this information still didn't seem to faze her.

The more Minnie insisted on returning to Florida, the more irritated I became. This time, I decided not to help her with the logistics of the move, or with the planning and packing.

I hoped that without my assistance she wouldn't be able to pull it off—but it didn't matter. Several chivalrous male residents toiled like slaves in return for Minnie's smiles and expressions of gratitude. Her charm had worked again.

I believed she was making a self-destructive mistake. She was becoming increasingly needy. Who would care for her in Florida? Try as I might to talk her out of it, my appeal fell on deaf ears.

I believed that she should be staying up north and I told her, often and forcefully. So did the social workers in her building.

"You really should stay," they told her. "Give yourself more time to adjust."

"I'm going back to Florida," she replied.

"You told me you hated Florida," I reminded her, "that you had nobody there anymore, and that your place was with your children."

"I'm going back to Florida," she replied. And she did. When Minnie made up her mind, she had a "whim of iron."

The relocation itself went off without a hitch. So, what to do? For starters, I called Gloria Gelman, our Florida social worker, to alert her to the return of the "prodigal Mom." Gloria was shocked and disappointed, but promised to contact Minnie as soon as she settled in.

Her goal, she told me after her first revisit to Minnie, was to convince Mom to move just one more time, this time into a congregate living facility in Florida, the kind that provided a continuum of accommodations for seniors; apartments for those that could live independently, and assisted living for those needing such support. Some of them even had skilled nursing beds on campus.

"Good luck," I said, liking the plan but doubting it was possible

"Leave it to me," Gloria said. "By the way," she said, "are you aware that your mother has leased a car, a little stripped down Toyota Corolla."

"What?" I exploded. "Who would lease a car to an elderly woman with obvious cognitive problems? How did this happen?" I was beside myself. "When did she do this? Why did she do this?"

"I sort of thought you didn't know," said Gloria. "She did it partially because she wants the independence of having a car. But mostly, in my opinion, she did it to spite you. You took away her car, so she's going to show you a thing or two. She asked me not to tell you about this, but I think she's secretly hoping that I do. Listen, Jerry, I've driven with her. In her hands, that little Toyota is a deadly weapon. Somehow, you have to get involved before she kills someone."

Weeks went by. I pondered and schemed. How could I get Minnie to stop driving without making her madder at me than she already was?

An idea! I called the Florida State Attorney General's office and suggested that Minnie's driver's license be pulled. The said they could do that only if I could prove she was a danger to the community.

When they checked her records, guess what. Minnie was a recipient of the State's "Careful Driver Award" for going twenty-five years without an accident. How could they cancel such a safe driver's license?

I explained that she didn't drive even once during the twenty-five years for which she earned the award, and I pointed out that it's hard to have an accident when you're not driving. It didn't matter. Minnie's license was safe.

It took some general, open-ended questions on my part, but Minnie finally, almost gleefully 'fessed up. It seems that a "very nice man she knew" referred her to a local dealer who persuaded this cognitively impaired widow to pay a large down payment and to sign a five-year lease for a car that retailed for about $11,000.

Mom's total cost for the car, after interest and fees, would be almost double that. A very profitable deal for the dealership, and probably for the "very nice man" who brought her in. Where were the consumer protection laws?

About a month later, out of the blue, Mom said, "Jerry, I want to get rid of the car."

Confused and exasperated, I replied, "Ma, you can't get rid of it. You signed a lease. It's a legal document. Why do you want to get rid of it?"

"I've decided to take an apartment at Happy Hollow."

"Happy Hollow?"

"Yeah. You should see it. It's in a beautiful setting. And they have swimming pools, recreation, meals, entertainment, you name it, and Jerry…"

"What?"

"They even have an assisted living section. Not that I need it, but you never know what the future will bring. And I won't need a car. They have transportation for their residents."

But "Happy Hollow?" Really, I wondered, where did they dream up these insipid names?

Surprised, but delighted by this unexpected turn of events, I said, "That's a terrific idea, Ma."

"I knew you'd approve," said Minnie. "I'm doing it for you so you can have peace of mind about me. It was Gloria's suggestion."

(Thank you Gloria!)

Minnie always needed to feel that whatever changes she made in her life were generous gifts she was giving to me. Somehow, it was contrary to her value system to ever do something just for herself. Oh well!

"It will give me peace of mind," I agreed and I added, "but you can't get rid of the car."

"What do you mean, I can't get rid of it? It's very expensive and I'll soon no longer need it. Jerry, you have to help to me give it back."

Remember, in Florida, many senior citizens made a practice of buying an item on Monday and returning it on Tuesday. Minnie fully expected to be able to do this with the car.

No matter how I tried to explain to her that you can't undo an auto lease without taking a financial bath, she just could not understand that she was stuck. She no longer wanted the car and it became my job to return it for a refund.

What could I do? I went into action.

First, I telephoned the dealer who said, as I expected, that nothing could be done. Minnie was over twenty-one and her signature on the car's purchase agreement was legal. It was hers.

The dealer had sold the "paper" to its financing subdivision. The latter also said that nothing could be done to undo the lease, but that Minnie could buy the car at the contract price.

It would cost her $18,000 to take ownership of the Toyota. This, plus her down payment, would mean that she would have spent over $20,000 for a cheap little car that she no longer wanted and that would only bring about $7,000 in the used car marketplace.

A $13,000 loss!

This would drastically deplete her dwindling cash resources. It was money she needed to support her day-to-day living.

I ranted and raved to the dealer about the immorality of this contract. It got me nowhere. Then I became obsessed. I flew to Florida and examined the car.

Other than the fact that it had been hugely overpriced, I could find nothing wrong with the Corolla. It drove nicely. Minnie had put all of 146 miles on it since she owned it, so it was like new. Remarkably, no sheet metal damage was evident. So far!

Next, I took Minnie to lawyers who promised to get her out of her lease, but their fees were outrageous. I contacted the Miami newspapers to suggest a special report on how auto dealerships were preying on the elderly. They told me they had done that special the previous month and were no longer interested in the issue.

I called the Florida Attorney General again. He listened politely but said that no laws were broken and he could do nothing. It was one dead end after another. So I went home to mull over the situation.

I was at my wit's end and becoming resigned to the financial impact when God stepped in. Now I'm not one who believes in a deity that concerns itself with every aspect of every living thing, or that gets involved in the minutia of our lives. Yet something does seem to look after the weakest among us.

It could have been just a coincidence, but I doubt it. Remarkably, Minnie was now my partner in trying to undo the car lease that she executed in her moment of pique. Suddenly, there was light at the end of the tunnel and it wasn't New Jersey.

Hope came in the form of a late night talk show. Minnie called in one morning at around 3 a.m., and explained the whole deal to the host (with whom she was now on a first name basis, God bless her).

The host understood an audience sympathy story when he heard one and he exploited it to the hilt. He soon became a strident broadcast advocate for Minnie against the dealership. The latter threatened to sue and the radio host threatened to counter sue.

The dealer collapsed first in this game of "chicken" and, amazingly, found a way to cancel this uncancellable lease. Minnie would be out her deposit, but that would be the extent of her pain providing that she returned the car within a week. In return, the radio host promised to stop badmouthing the dealership and to give it some free plugs on the air.

Thus, there was a win/win for everyone...except, of course, for the future elderly victims of this dealer's unsavory sales practices.

But Minnie was off the hook. She asked me to come down again over the weekend to help get the car ready to turn in. I wasn't clear on why she needed me, but I had an uncomfortable feeling and agreed to come.

I arrived on a Friday evening. The Corolla was due at the dealership on Monday and had to be in tiptop shape. One look at the car and my adrenalin started to pump. You guessed it. Bent fenders were everywhere.

There goes this deal, I thought. Would it be possible to get the body repaired on a Saturday or Sunday with the kind of quality needed to pass the dealer's inspection on Monday? Again, my heart sank.

It needn't have. Where I live, this would have been an impossible task, but this was Florida, the land of the senior citizen driver.

I checked the yellow pages and discovered that, in Minnie's little town alone, there were hundreds of auto body shops. Ditto for each of the neighboring towns. And all of the shops were open for business on the weekend and anxious to compete for the work on the Corolla.

Who would have believed it? On Monday, looking as good as new, the car was successfully returned and the nightmare was over.

Minnie never drove again and, for a while anyway, she seemed to have forgiven me. Our relationship was again cordial. But many "adventures" remained in Minnie Sweet's long, slow decline into dementia.

A HAPPY HOLLOWGRAM

So Minnie's condo was finally sold. This time, there was no turning back for her and she was once again on the move. Her destination: the Happy Hollow Residence for seniors.

Everything that had been jammed into her double storage bins at the condo somehow fit into the single large basement storage cage that she was allotted at Happy Hollow.

And here was something new. Since she gave much of her stuff to her grandchildren during her in-and-out gambit to "live near her children" in Michigan, all of her remaining furniture could be accommodated in her new apartment. It was tight but livable.

For the moment, she was actually happy and, as long as I didn't have to retrieve anything from storage, so was I.

The place was as lovely as she had described, and Gloria Gelman vouched for its reputation. The monthly rent was expensive but, when you considered Minnie's potential savings in food, utility and similar costs, it was not unreasonable.

Also, while she didn't quite recoup her investment on the sale of her condo, she came close, and the proceeds gave her savings balance a much needed infusion of capital.

Amazingly, she finally agreed to share some information with me about the state of her assets. Although she still would not let me manage them, I could now realistically estimate the length of time that her money might last.

My calculations indicated that she should be able to support her needs for about five more years…that is providing she didn't lease any more cars or engage in similar antics. What if she lived longer? That was to be hoped for and to be faced at the time.

She was having more and more difficulty coping with her checkbook, her certificates of deposit, and her bills. Whenever I was with her she invariably pulled dozens of envelopes from her drawers and from her dresser top (which was getting to be as cluttered with paper as her previous residences had been).

"Look at these things," she would say and then go on to ask, "Jerry, which ones are important?"

It was obvious that she was becoming increasingly confused. At first I thought it was her eyesight that was deteriorating, but a trip to the optometrist eliminated that theory. It was her cognition.

Many of the envelopes she showed me contained advertising or were otherwise what you would call "junk mail." Buried among these useless mailings were always several real bills, or correspondence dealing with banking, legal or insurance issues. Minnie could no longer tell the difference.

This scared me. I recalled how my father handled his mother's affairs as she aged. It took a lot of his time and energy, for which he received little thanks and much criticism from Mme. Sweet.

Other caregivers told me horror stories about aged parents with dementia that paid some of their bills multiple times and others not at all.

Though I really didn't need the headache, I decided that I should more frequently and forcefully offer to provide bookkeeping service for Minnie. Sooner or later, I thought, reality would force her to delegate this.

Here's how the conversation would go when I was with her following one of these reviews of her "in-box."

"Ma, are you ready to have me manage your finances?"

"Absolutely, Jerry. I'd like that. How can we do this?"

"Well, Ma, it means that I would have to be a signer on your bank accounts and that all your mail would be forwarded to me up north."

"All my mail? What about letters and greeting cards from my friends and family?"

"No problem. I would only ask your billers to do this. Personal mail would still go directly to you."

"Jerry, let me think about it, but it may be a good idea. Call me when you get home and let's talk about it some more."

Each time I returned home, however, whenever I raised the topic by phone, the conversation went like this:

"Ma, how are you doing with your mail and your bills?"

"Fine."

"Do you still want me to handle this for you."

"No."

"Ma, I'm worried about you. I thought you agreed that it was becoming a burden for you. I'd be happy to relieve you of it."

"Jerry, everyone here says I shouldn't do it."

"Everyone? Okay, you say 'everyone,' so let's accept that for the moment, but why? Does 'everyone' have a good reason?"

"Everyone has a story of how someone's kids stole all their money. I know you wouldn't do that, but I think I'll do my own finances for a while longer. Okay?"

"Of course, it's okay," I'd say, not really blaming her. When she gave up her car she lost a huge part of her sense of independence. Giving up control of her money represented an even bigger threat.

I didn't take it personally, but I worried about her shrinking resources and whether she knew how to make her assets last.

At one point, she chuckled and admitted that she couldn't make any sense of her checkbook balance anymore, and she decided to allow me to balance it monthly. That was a revelation.

I went back as far as the date that Sidney died and could not recreate a complete trail of deposits and checks. For several years, many items had not been entered in the checkbook. Numerous bank statements, including some recent ones, were missing. So it was impossible to accurately balance her books.

Still, it gave me some idea of how she was spending her money and, with a little bit of creative accounting, I found I was able to reconcile her account within a comfortable range.

This went on for about a year when, somehow, she misplaced a Social Security check, probably throwing it out. The check was ultimately replaced by the feds, but this experience frightened her, big time, and she almost came around on this issue.

She decided to add my signature authority to all of her assets, "just in case" something happened to her but, for better or worse, she remained adamant about controlling her own finances.

Meanwhile, the issues were beginning to mount up. For example, she was becoming socially isolated. While she made lots of acquaintances at Happy Hollow, there was nobody close.

She said that she wasn't able to "bond" with anyone there—a strange new condition for this formerly outgoing people person.

Also, she was becoming incontinent. Upon entering her apartment, the smell of urine was subtle but unmistakable. "Accidents" were not unusual for someone her age but, if this was happening to Minnie, someone needed to approach her about it. How could I do this without embarrassing her?

I couldn't, I decided, and I called in the Mounties in the form of Minnie's sister, my aunt Charlotte. What she learned was that Minnie was indeed having what she called some "leakage," but that she felt ashamed and was unwilling to use any of the absorbent pads available in every drugstore for this purpose.

She was changing her panties a lot and stuffing them in the laundry basket where they became malodorous awaiting the weekly pick up. Our conclusion: this was another sign of accelerating decline, but it wasn't yet serious enough to make it a major concern.

Her hallucination about mice—the belief that hundreds of the little rodents infested her condo and my home up north—was transferred to her new apartment.

She also suffered from a lifelong abhorrence of cats. The widow in the next apartment owned one that was terrorizing Minnie. Actually, all the little feline did was lick its paws and lie harmlessly in the sun near the window at the end of the corridor—but Minnie was convinced the lady was letting it out to spite her.

"Ma," I joked, "it's a good thing, isn't it? The cat can take care of your mouse problem."

She didn't see the humor. All she did was glare at me in silence, and I immediately regretted my comment.

The Administrator at Happy Hollow referred to Minnie's emotional cycles...periods when she seemed agitated and unhappy and verbally abusive of everyone, followed by periods of gentle tranquility.

"Nothing they couldn't handle," he said, but something he felt I needed to know about.

She was taking her dinners in the dining room, but her refrigerator was almost bare except for some moldy cheese. I wondered what she was eating for breakfast and lunch.

She was quite overweight, so she had to be eating something...but was Minnie eating healthily? I resolved to find out, but questioning her about it was unproductive, and her health seemed to be getting worse.

In recent months, Minnie had been hospitalized several times for pneumonia. She was diagnosed with

COPD (Chronic Obstructive Pulmonary Disease). And she spent two weeks in an inpatient program for people with crippling arthritis, something that nobody but Minnie thought she had.

She somehow managed to badger her doctor into ordering this so the Medicare HMO would pay for it. For him, the path of least resistance was to quietly accept her self-diagnosis.

Minnie was visiting the doctor more frequently, but not taking her prescribed medications because of side effects imagined or real...or maybe she was just forgetting?

Her doctor was affiliated with Happy Hollow. He maintained regular office hours there, and he was connected to her latest HMO.

The good news was that Minnie was seeing him and she liked him. That bode well for continuity in her care. Even though I had some concerns about his credentials in geriatrics, I was not going to do anything to cause Minnie to resume her old pattern of doctor hopping.

The bad news was that this doctor was not particularly fluent in English or openly communicative with patients or family members.

It hardly mattered what I thought, though, since her choice of primary doctors and specialists was limited to the approved panel in her HMO, none of whom, in my opinion, were likely to be any more qualified than this Happy Hollow physician and his referral network.

Once, when I sought out her doctor to mention my suspicion that Minnie had the beginnings of a dementia, he related that it wasn't merely a "beginning." In his opinion, she was well down the road and would soon need assisted living

"It will only get worse, you know," he said, "so you better be prepared."

If I hadn't asked, I don't think he was planning to tell me this. Having told me, however, he decided to recommend that Minnie see a psychiatrist to evaluate whether her behavior was dementia-related or due to some other psychiatric disorder.

I felt good about this until I discovered that the psychiatrist spoke little English and had no understanding of Minnie's ethnic and cultural background. This did little to give me confidence in the results of his evaluation.

In fairness, I have to say that the medications the psychiatrist prescribed did seem to improve her attitude and her interpersonal relationships a bit…that is when she remembered to take them.

His conclusion was that Minnie had multiple problems—dementia, anxiety disorder, and a mild psychosis typical of patients at her stage. He also suggested that she be moved to the assisted living section of Happy Hollow.

Gloria Gelman, who remained in the picture at my request, agreed with him about Minnie's need for a more structured setting. But Minnie resisted this idea with all her strength.

I could no longer deny that my mother was sinking deeper into a fog with each passing day—that her aggravating behavior and growing deficits were leading her down a slippery slope.

Years earlier, the same thing happened to Minnie's mother and her older sister, so I shouldn't have been surprised—but I was. It was not Alzheimer's but a dementia with a multi-infarct etiology.

The diagnosis was less important to me, however, than the reality of her disease. I was learning to accept the fact that I was not seeing the real Minnie. I was seeing her illness.

For the first time, I began to really grieve. In some ways, coping with my mother's dementia was worse for me than the shock I felt with Sidney's sudden exit.

I grieved for Sidney for about a year, during which the intensity of my loss lessened with each month that passed. With dementia, on the other hand, one grieves all the time.

You realize that your parent is no longer intact and you grieve. Then you grow accustomed to the way she is and stop grieving until the next decline in her competence and in her ability to manage. At that point, you feel like you have lost her again and you start to grieve anew.

This scenario then repeats itself over and over and over and, if your loved one lives a long time, like Minnie, it feels like she has died over and over and over.

At this writing, Sidney has been gone almost fifteen years and, with perfect hindsight, I can now date Minnie's decline to at least a year prior to that event. But that's looking backward.

Day to day, one hardly notices the change. Only when comparing her today with the way she was one, two, five, or ten years ago, does the extent of her decline become apparent.

A friend suggested a book entitled the "36-Hour Day," by Nancy L. Mace, M.A., and Peter V. Rabins, M.D., M.P.H., published by the Johns Hopkins University Press.

This book changed my entire perspective about Minnie's situation and enabled me to feel sympathy and empathy for her for the first time in years...and to understand that I was not alone in dealing with the personality changes and erratic conduct of an aging parent. I highly recommend it to anyone coping with a dementia in a loved one.

But let's get back to our chronological narrative.

Minnie, of course, continued to resist moving to the assisted living program at Happy Hollow until an accident forced her to change her mind.

A phone call from the Administrator interrupted my business day. He reported that a security guard found Minnie lying on the floor, unconscious and in her own excrement.

She apparently lost her balance and remained in the spot where she fell for over 24 hours. There was a nasty bump on the back of her head, and she had to be admitted to a hospital. There was no need for me to fly down, he said.

The lump was caused by a hematoma, but she was otherwise all right. He said that she could continue to live at Happy Hollow, but that she would have to move to assisted living. In his opinion, she could no longer live safely in an independent apartment.

"Are you telling me that she doesn't have a choice?" I asked. "If she wants to stay at Happy Hollow, she must make the move?"

"That's what I'm telling you," he said. "Its for her own protection."

I flew down anyway and had to agree that, aside from the bump on her head, Minnie seemed physically okay. Mentally was another story.

She didn't remember anything about the fall, or being in the hospital for that matter, but she agreed to move to assisted living in order (of course) to give me peace of mind.

She also asked me to take over the day-to-day handling of her financial affairs.

Dementia Diary

RESISTED LIVING

.

"Jerry, you have to get me out of this place."

Minnie sounded agitated on the phone and my spirits sank listening to her. For her sake, and mine, I hoped she would quickly adjust and be happy in her new assisted living digs.

But this was Minnie we were talking about, the lady who ran back to Florida less than two months after her "permanent" move up north. Adjustment was for other people. Minnie expected perfect, every time.

"You just moved in. What's wrong, Ma?"

"They steal here, that's what's wrong."

"Really? That is serious. Are you sure?"

"Did you ever know me to lie, Jerry? Of course I'm sure."

"I know you wouldn't make something like that up, Ma, but couldn't you be mistaken? Is something of yours missing?"

"I'm not mistaken. They took my small vacuum cleaner, you know, the one that operates on batteries, and they took my dishes and tableware. I have nothing to eat with because they took it."

"Calm down, Ma. Who do you mean by 'they'?"

"The help here, Jerry. You can't turn your back."

"Listen, Ma. The vacuum and tableware are in your basement storage cages. I put them there myself. You get all your meals in the assisted living program and are not even permitted to cook or eat anything in your room except, maybe, a light snack now and then. Nobody stole these things."

"Oh yeah, Mr. Wise Guy, what about my wedding ring, the one with the diamonds that your father bought me for our fiftieth? If nobody's stealing, what happened to that?"

"The ring is missing?"

"The ring is missing. They took it when I wasn't in the room."

"And what would you be doing leaving a ring like that visible in the room when you were out?"

"Jerry," she shouted, near hysteria now, "it's gone and they took it. You have to get it back."

"Okay, Ma. Okay. I'll see what I can do. Did you report it to the Administrator."

"He's probably in on it. Jerry, get me my ring back or I'm leaving this place."

Oy! Could someone have stolen her diamond wedding band? I thought it possible, but not likely. Minnie sounded almost irrational about it. Still, it could have happened. I decided to call the Administrator.

"They all have these delusions," he said.

"What do you mean?" I asked, feeling a bit hostile at his flip attitude.

"Don't get me wrong, Mr. Sweet. I don't mean to minimize the problem, or insult your mother. But dementia does strange things to perception and memory. I really doubt that anyone stole it. It would be too easy to identify the culprit."

"You mean you never have a problem with theft by your staff?"

"Of course, we have. Every facility like ours has such incidents. It's just that the number of real thefts is a tiny percentage of the claims by residents. Look, I'll check it out. Don't worry. Unless the ring went down the sink or toilet, and believe me that happens a lot here, I bet it will turn up exactly where she put it for safekeeping."

Several days later, Minnie herself found the ring. It was wrapped in a wad of tissue paper and stuffed into a small plastic purse that was stuffed into a larger plastic purse that was stuffed into an even larger leather purse that was stuffed into the back of one of her dresser drawers.

When she called to tell me about it, I asked, "So, are you satisfied now that no one is stealing?"

"I know what they're doing, Jerry. You scared them by calling the Administrator. Whoever took the ring put it back when I wasn't looking."

"Ma, that's ridiculous. You put it there yourself and don't want to admit it."

"Oh yeah? Well what about my sunglasses?"

"What about your sunglasses?"

"Somebody stole them."

"Were they prescription sunglasses?"

"They were."

"Ma, why would anyone steal prescription sunglasses? That doesn't make any sense. You're the only one who can use them."

And so the conversation went. For weeks, things were missing only to be found shortly afterwards where, I am certain, Minnie put them. I believe she felt foolish each time the missing item reappeared in one of her pockets or drawers, but she was too embarrassed to confess her role in the problem.

The good news was that she stopped threatening to move. So I knew that no one was really stealing anything of hers, and I knew that she knew it too.

For a few months she seemed to be more content. I began to relax and even thought that she was adjusting nicely to the new arrangement. But that was not to last.

There was twenty-four hour nursing coverage…well, not real nurses, mostly aides from Haiti…but they were very caring and there was an actual RN in charge of the daytime shift. Among other things, they were responsible for giving Minnie her prescription medications, and what a difference that made.

Her medication cocktail included anti-depressants, anti-anxiety, and antipsychotic drugs, as well as pills for her digestive and urinary symptoms. Now that she was taking these meds on schedule, you could hear the improvement in her telephone voice. She sounded calmer and less bitter. You might even say happy.

"Ma," I said, expecting the usual complaints, "how do you like your new situation?"

"It's very nice, Jerry. I'm getting used to it."

"You actually seem happy, Ma. I'm so pleased."

"Happy? Who said anything about 'happy'? I said I'm getting used to it. What has that got to do with 'happy'?"

Oops! I forgot. It was against Minnie's instincts and upbringing to allow her son to think she was happy. Better not to mention it, even if she did seem more cheerful.

"I just meant that you seem to be recovering from that bad fall you took in the apartment. I feel much relieved that someone is always available to you and keeping an eye on you. I wouldn't want you to hurt yourself again and to have to wait two days for help. Don't you feel more secure now?"

"You're right, Jerry. I do feel safer, and I wouldn't want you to worry. So, I'll make the best of it here."

Make the best of it? Her enthusiasm was "whelming."

"Another thing, Ma," I said, ignoring her last jibe, "I think the medications you take are helping you."

"What medications? I'm not taking anything?"

"Yes you are. Your nurses told me the names of the drugs you are taking and that they are really working."

"They're lying, Jerry. I'd know if I was taking drugs, and I'm not."

She was becoming agitated by my questions, so I decided to change the subject.

"Whatever you say, Ma. I'm sure you know what you're taking. Listen, how's the food in the new dining room."

"Terrible."

"Sorry to hear that. 'Bye, Ma."

"'Bye, Jerry."

There was no point in pursuing the food question. The biggest item of complaint in facilities like Happy Hollow is the food. Institutional food, no matter how well prepared, is still institutional food. Monotonous and, usually, cheap. Nourishing, but cheap.

Still, the food problem refused to go away. Every time Minnie and I talked, it came up and, soon, it became the major topic in our conversations. Something else was going on and it wasn't just about food. But what? I decided to fly down and see. Nadine came with me.

What we discovered was that there was a caste system at Happy Hollow. Minnie's original apartment was in the "Independent Living" section. For these residents, there was a large, luxurious dining room with a selective menu.

People in "Assisted Living," on the other hand, were assigned to a segregated dining room with a restrictive menu. They were not permitted to eat in the main dining room.

Many assisted living residents were very far along in their dementias and, for them, the arrangement made sense. Minnie's condition, however, was borderline at that time, and for her it was an oppressive and offensive system.

When Minnie moved to assisted living at Happy Hollow, her social standing dropped several notches. People that she previously mingled with in the independent living dining room were treating her like she had the plague. She was now one of "those people."

To make matters worse, she tried several times to eat in the main dining room but was refused service. She was stigmatized, yet was still sound enough, mentally and emotionally, to sustain a major hurt because of this.

I intervened forcefully with the Administrator and got permission for Minnie to eat in the main dining room whenever she had company, but this was too little, too late. I couldn't blame my mother for wanting out, and out she wanted.

My only question was "where to next?"

Minnie's answer: "My place is with my children."

Been there! Done that!

"You can't be serious, Ma," I said. "Think about what happened last time. I don't have the emotional strength, and you don't have enough money, to do a reprise."

"What do you mean?"

"Ma, it's less than two years since you moved up to us the first time. You were so unhappy that you lasted only two months before you returned to Florida. We can't put you through that again...and we definitely can't put me through that again."

"I did that?"

"Don't tell me you don't remember."

Silence. Her eyes glazed. She looked really confused, then suddenly focused again. Finally, "It's time Jerry. Maybe I wasn't ready then. Now I'm ready."

I began to think that maybe she really didn't have a clear recollection of the disaster of her last attempt to relocate up north.

"Tell you what," I said, against my better judgment. "I'm coming down for another visit next month. Let's think it over and talk about it then. If you really mean it, let's consider it, but Ma…"

"What?"

"If you do it, you have to make a commitment. It has to be permanent. You must give yourself adjustment time, and there'll be no going back."

"Okay. But I won't change my mind."

With my head spinning, and every muscle of my body in "fight or flight" mode, I changed the subject to one of her favorites. It was time for an organ recital.

"Tell me, Ma," I asked, "how have you been feeling?"

It was a perfect distraction. Minnie easily shifted from obsessing about her latest whim (that is, torturing me by asking to move north again), to a complete rundown of all of her bodily systems.

As usual, she went into much greater detail than is necessary to report here. What you need to know, though, is that she did have some major health issues in addition to her imaginary ones.

She had recently been hospitalized several times with repeated episodes of pneumonia, and was thought to have a condition known as COPD (Chronic Obstructive Pulmonary Disease).

Her growing daily drug list now included "puffs," a cute word for those pressurized steroid inhalants that have become so common among people of all ages with pulmonary problems.

Here's another sign of Minnie's slipping abilities. I watched the nursing aides try to administer these medications, and it was clear that Minnie couldn't coordinate taking a breath with the intake of the puff. She was like a child.

After the drug was administered, instead of inhaling, she would open her mouth, and out would seep the dose that should have gone into her lungs. It took many tries to medicate her adequately.

Also, she had constant pain in her back and, more worrisome, in her leg. Walking had become so difficult for her that she rarely left her room, except to limp down the hall at mealtimes. I decided to talk to her doctor.

"Arthritis," the doctor said.

"Are you sure? Maybe you should do some tests or take some x-rays. What if it's something more serious?"

"It's nothing to worry about. It's just arthritis. I see it all the time. More tests will just be expensive and they aren't justified by your mother's condition. But trust me, it's normal at her age."

Remember these words. The leg will come up again in a later chapter.

Before Nadine and I flew back up north, we decided to take Minnie on an outing to the seashore. It was something she hadn't done in years, even though the ocean was only ten minutes away. She was thrilled.

However, walking the short distance from the car to the beach was painful and it exhausted her. She had to sit down on a blanket in the sand where she decided to remain while my wife and I took a walk along the surf. Minnie didn't have the energy to join us.

When we retrieved her, I was startled by two pieces of reality. One, she could not rise from the sitting position without major assistance and, more disturbing, her hand was shaking with a kind of jerky palsy.

Minnie called my attention to this with a detached curiosity, as though the hand belonged to someone else, but I was devastated. I had been in deep denial about my mother's deteriorating physical condition. Clearly, it was no longer possible for me to do this.

Home again, barely a week had passed when the lobbying began in earnest. I was in the office trying to catch up with my workload when the first of many such calls from Minnie came in. I've kind of compressed them into a single conversation, as follows:

"Jerry, I've done what you asked."

"That's nice, Ma. What about?" As if I didn't know.

"You know. About my coming to live near you."

"I thought we agreed to just think about it for awhile."

"That's what I mean. I have thought about it. My place is with my children."

There's that phrase again. It was starting to wear on me. "You mean you want to move in with Nadine and me?" My fingers were crossed.

"Absolutely not. I never wanted to be a burden to you, and I'll not start now."

Phew! So what was an only son to do? I love my mother and wanted her to have a safe and comfortable old age. However, she was doing an increasing number of erratic things, and was arguing with me continually over just about everything. Every phone call ended in a screaming match.

Also, people were telling us that Minnie was criticizing Nadine and me to anyone who would listen (except to our faces, when she would emote endlessly about how "wonderful" we were), and she was just about driving me crazy.

I've only had room to describe a fraction of the many colorful (read aggravating) incidents that she precipitated, but there's no need for me to document them all. You get the idea. If you've read this far, you know enough about what "Managing Minnie" has been like since Sidney died.

Even though I knew, intellectually, that Minnie's behavior was a manifestation of her illness, I was having a harder and harder time dealing with it emotionally. The thought of having the source of these pressures living nearby was terrifying.

On the other hand, as Minnie got older and frailer, I knew I'd have to be commuting to Florida constantly, disrupting my life and livelihood in the process, to see first hand what I would not be able to assess long distance. It was a toss up as to which option was least desirable.

This was one of the times that I anticipated when I engaged Gloria Gelman's services way back when all this started. More than ever before, I needed someone objective to help me analyze my choices.

I wanted to do the right thing for Minnie, but I also wanted to do the right thing for Nadine and me. It was time to consult my Super Social Worker.

"Hello, Gloria."

"Hi Jerry."

Gloria walked me through the pros and cons of my alternatives. In typical social work fashion, she didn't come right out and say what she thought I should do, but she asked penetrating questions that enabled me to think through my dilemma.

Although she never said so, I had the distinct impression from her questions that she would favor moving Minnie up.

Actually, it was Nadine who helped me make the decision. "Do whatever feels right to you," she said. "These are Minnie's last years. Make sure that when she dies, you won't have any regrets about the choices you make now."

That did it. "Ma," I said when she answered the phone. "Have you thought about where you would live if you moved up here?"

"No. I'll go wherever you say."

"What about that Senior Residence that you and Dad looked at once when you were both visiting us?"

There was no way that Sidney would have agreed to live in such a facility, but Minnie seemed to like it. It's actually a licensed home for the aged but, for marketing reasons, it has another name that's more acceptable to aging residents who think negative thoughts about homes for the aged.

At the time of Minnie's campaign to get me to agree to this relocation, it was evolving into an assisted living program where people would be permitted to age in place. I thought it would be a perfect fit for her at this time in her life. From now on, I will refer to it simply as the "Residence."

"I don't remember it Jerry, but if you say it's the right place, that's good enough for me."

"I don't know if they have any vacancies, Ma. There might be a waiting list. Do you want me to find out?"

And that's how the "boomerang bubbe" came full circle once again. When Sidney died she was seventy-seven. She was now eighty-three years old.

NORTHWARD HO

Here's how the second relocation north went. In order to avoid some of the issues that plagued Minnie's previous moves, I knew I had to get rid of as much of her stuff as possible.

For years, she hoarded all kinds of things, and her room was jammed with tchatchkes (that's Yiddish for decorative things having little monetary value and even less practical utility). Her basement storage cage was even more of a problem.

In discussing these things Minnie, at first, seemed agreeable to my helping her decide what to keep and what to discard. Nevertheless, on the day in question, she reverted to her norm and began throwing her body, arms extended protectively, over anything that I tried to mark for charity or discard.

I understood that she was just trying to protect the remains of her active life and her memories. However, understanding and compassion did not change my practical need to complete the job. It was heartbreaking work. I literally had to peel her off everything that needed to be tossed.

This would never do. It was a Saturday and, of course, the movers were expected first thing Monday morning. Fortunately, Minnie's sister, my Aunt Charlotte again came to the rescue. She understood what was happening and invited Minnie to spend her last two days in Florida at Charlotte's apartment.

"They asked me to stay with them," Minnie said.

They, I thought? "Who are 'they'?" I asked.

Minnie looked puzzled by my question. "You know...'them'...I often stay with them."

"But," I protested, "it was Charlotte who invited you and she lives alone."

She smiled. "That's right. That's what I said. I'll go to Charlotte's place—I'd like to go now if that's okay."

I didn't say anything for a moment. Could Mom be having pronoun confusion... using the plural form when the singular was needed? If so, was it yet another early warning sign of something slipping inside her head?

Could she be saying "they" and "them" when she really meant "she" and "her"? And even more startling, could she not be aware of doing this? Yes...yes...and yes.

Strangely, though, she only did it at first when referring to her sister. I decided not to call her attention to this odd speech anomaly. It would just upset her.

It was to happen over and over again in the years ahead, would gradually worsen, and would ultimately lead to a serious aphasia...the loss of her ability to speak, write, or comprehend the meaning of many spoken or written words. But that horror was still several years in the future.

"Of course, it's okay," I said, trying not to sound too eager.

"Are you really sure you don't mind?" she asked. "This is a lot of work for you to do alone."

"No problem, Ma…but do you feel comfortable with me making all the decisions about what to keep and what to throw out?"

She thought about this for a while, but then consented to delegate the task. I think she was relieved to be spared the decision making process. Each item represented a nostalgic treasure. It was too much for her, and I drove her over to Charlotte's.

I felt certain that I would have a free hand to do what I wanted with all of her stuff, and that this was a golden opportunity to finally get rid of all kinds of junk. Her memory being what it was, I was convinced that she would never notice what was missing, and I turned out to be right. Out of sight, out of mind.

The problem turned out not to be Minnie, but me. As I went through her things all Saturday and Sunday, I did so through my tears.

There were my father's golf trophies, some of their many plaques for community service, clothes that wouldn't be appropriate up north, and all sorts of things that weren't essential, but which were part of Minnie and Sidney's household for decades.

Some items I even remembered fondly from my childhood. I just steeled myself and did what had to be done.

Late Sunday, a relative of Nadine's who ran a nearby flea market came with a truck and carted off all of the discards that might find a buyer. The rest went into the dumpster.

I felt like a traitor and all weekend, whenever I returned to Charlotte's place, I could hardly bring myself to make eye contact with Minnie.

Anyway, as usual, Monday morning arrived on schedule. The movers quickly loaded the rest of Minnie's goods and, by that evening, she was up north in an airport wheelchair waiting for me to bring the car around to take her to our house.

She was planning to spend one night with us, and be admitted to the Residence the following morning. So far, things had gone more smoothly than I had any right to expect.

But on Tuesday morning she panicked. She was seized by an anxiety attack so powerful that nothing could calm her. Essentially, Minnie announced that she was not going to the Residence, and that was that. I begged, pleaded, reasoned, ordered, all to no avail. She was not going anywhere.

"Ma, please. You wanted this."

Nothing.

"So what do you want to do?" I tried again.

"I'll stay with you. You have room. I'll just stay here."

"You're welcome to, Ma, but I thought you didn't want to be a burden. Anyway, it's not a good idea. Nadine and I are not home all day. We are out many times at night too, and we travel a lot. You can't be alone all that time, can you?"

Face flushed. Hands tightly clasped into fists. Knuckles white.

"I'll go back to Florida."

"Where to? You can't go back to Happy Hollow. You have no place to live in Florida."

"I'll stay with Charlotte."

"You know that Charlotte only lives there during the winters. She's leaving soon and you can't stay there alone either."

"I'll stay with the Stromberg's."

When Sidney died, Mark and Anna Stromberg offered to do anything Minnie needed to help her recover from being plunged into widowhood. They had been close friends for decades, and they all lived in the same retirement complex.

Unfortunately, less than a month after Sidney's funeral, Mark had a massive stroke. He survived, but lost all speech and mobility. It was an awful tragedy and Anna took it badly. Suddenly, the Stromberg's needed at least as much support as Minnie did.

The only problem from Minnie's point of view was that Anna did not stop talking about her bad luck. Two emotionally needy women, long time friends, were now competing for sympathy from each other, and from all the other people they had in common.

So Minnie, already in the early stages of her dementia, began to badmouth Anna and to avoid her.

I was shocked by my mother's lack of compassion for friends of so many years, and for the negative things that she had to say about them.

In retrospect, it was most likely her fear and her disease speaking, not the loving and generous mother who raised me. But, at the time, it really disturbed me.

Now, six years after Mark Stromberg's stroke, Minnie was sitting stubbornly in my living room, arms crossed and teeth clenched. She had conveniently forgotten the callous way she had rejected the Stromberg's. All she could think of was their wonderful offer at Sidney's funeral to help her in her time of need.

And all I could think of was her unsuccessful attempt, several years back, to get me to promise not to "put her" in a nursing home.

True, the Residence Minnie was heading for was not a nursing home, and since she had freely chosen it, I was not "putting her" there. Still, I felt there were symbolic similarities to the thing Minnie feared about nursing homes, even if she was not consciously aware of it at the moment.

Talk about guilt, I felt like I'd cornered the market on that emotion. In any event, whatever Minnie was thinking, the Stromberg option was an out-of-the-question fantasy, and I needed to get that across to her.

"Ma, Anna has her hands full with caring for Mark. She doesn't need a boarder."

Minnie looked genuinely puzzled. I gently reminded her of her recent history with the Stromberg's and her face softened.

"I did that?" she said.

"Yes."

"Mark had a stroke?"

"Yes."

"Jerry, I don't remember."

"I know."

The storm was over. Minnie had become docile and rational and put up no further resistance to keeping her admission appointment that morning at the Residence.

The first thing she saw upon arrival was a group of the oldest and weakest residents sitting around in the lobby surrounded by walkers and wheelchairs. Some were alert, but many were sleeping in their seats.

"Look at them, Jerry. I don't belong here."

"This is only a few of the residents, Ma. There are a lot of people like you here. Give it a chance."

"Okay, but I'm only doing it for you."

"Fine!"

The situation reminded me of the time during Sidney's Shiva (the mourning period immediately following a death in a Jewish family) when Minnie threw a guest with Alzheimer's out of her house.

Many people were visiting, talking about Sidney's positive attributes, and sharing snacks in accordance with custom.

First, let's talk about those snacks. There were platters of cold cuts that Nadine and I purchased to feed the expected visitors. As the people arrived to pay their respects, Nadine and Aunt Charlotte tried to bring the food out of the kitchen.

Suddenly, Minnie became very agitated and blocked the platters with her body.

"What are you doing?" Charlotte asked. "All these people are here to show their compassion and empathy for you. We have to serve them. "

"No we don't," shouted Minnie, her face red with anger. "Those people don't care a bit about me or Sidney. They just came here for the food, and I don't want them to have it."

It took a full half hour of Charlotte's most skillful diplomacy to get Minnie to back off and permit the food to be served.

Actually, it wasn't only the diplomacy. She was distracted by something else, something that made her even more upset and irrational than the cold cuts.

Here's what it was—a cousin of Nadine's had arrived to express her condolences, and she had brought her mother along in a wheelchair.

Minnie took one look and, rather than being gracious and appreciative of the sentiments involved, she loudly insisted that "that woman with the Alzheimer's" be removed from her home at once.

I believe that Minnie understood viscerally that the woman in the wheelchair represented her future, and that in rejecting the person she was somehow defeating the inevitable.

To this day, Nadine's cousin has been forgiving and understanding of what probably was a feeling of apprehension so powerful that Minnie could not prevent her anti-social reaction.

I can't explain her behavior with the cold cuts, except to note it as part of a growing pattern. I don't know whether she had any conscious inkling of her own early cognitive losses, but I certainly did not as yet. I just felt mortified by her behavior.

But that was then and this was now. I needn't have worried. The rest of the admission process to the Residence went well. The movers arrived and loaded up her room, but Minnie had changed. Some of the old fire was gone.

She barely protested when Nadine and I said we were taking many of the cartons home with us to store for her in our basement. More surprisingly, she did not object when we suggested offering some of her furnishings to staff members at the Residence.

As much as I appreciated her cooperation, I missed her old assertiveness and felt a sense of loss. Was this my mother?

Of all the mountains of possessions that had crammed her previous lodgings, all that was left in her new one-room apartment was her own dresser and mirror, one bedside table, a couple of lamps, a portable black and white TV that she seldom watched, half a dozen plaques (out of a possible fifty or so), and a much reduced assortment of family photos to be hung on her walls.

She even turned over guardianship of some valuable jewelry to Nadine for fear of losing it or having it stolen. Other than the modest clothing wardrobe we placed in her closet and her dresser drawers, plus some books and costume jewelry, that was it.

The first serious problem she faced in her new world was the chronic and constant pain in her leg. It had never gone away.

We needed to make arrangements for Minnie's medical care and soon discovered that an internist with an interest in Geriatrics held office hours every Wednesday on the premises of the Residence.

"Your mother can hardly walk," said the doctor.

This was addressed to me. Minnie was sitting there looking very blank.

"I know," I replied. It's her arthritis."

"Who told you that?"

"Her doctor in Florida."

This elicited some mumbled comments, among which I thought I heard words like "incompetence," "stupidity," and similar epithets. They were articulated softly, so I couldn't be certain.

What I did hear the doctor say audibly was, "I doubt that it's arthritis."

"Really? What do you think it is?"

"A blood clot"

"A blood clot? Isn't that dangerous?"

"Yes, of course. If I'm right, Minnie runs a risk of 'throwing a clot' at any moment. That could be fatal, or cause a debilitating stroke."

My spirits fell but, somehow, I wasn't surprised. "What should we do?"

"I'm referring her to an excellent cardiologist for a complete workup. Do it soon. As I say, this is very dangerous."

Turning to Minnie, the doctor added, "Mrs. Sweet, do you understand what I'm telling your son?"

Minnie smiled and nodded, but it was clear that she didn't.

It turned out that it was a large blood clot and it was only dumb luck that it didn't kill her while she lived at Happy Hollow. Speaking of killing, Minnie's Florida physician was lucky I could not get my hands on him.

What followed was an awful week in the hospital where Minnie received massive blood thinning medication in order to dissolve the clot.

She was anguished and confused during the entire experience. She was in a two-bed room with a dying patient as a neighbor, a woman who groaned painfully twenty-four hours a day.

After a time, Minnie started bruising extensively from minor bumps, and the blood thinner had to be reduced. But the danger was over and, best of all, she could walk without pain for the first time in almost a year.

"Isn't this pretty basic medicine?" I asked the doctor.

"Of course."

"How could a licensed physician confuse a blood clot with arthritis?"

"Just be happy we found it and dissolved it. Forget about the rest." was the reply.

And this made sense. There was nothing I could do about the past, but Minnie now had access to much higher quality medical services than were available to her at Happy Hollow.

This was indeed something to be happy about. I've only been talking about the delivery of service, however. Paying for it was something else.

That part of the deal could be entitled, "The war of the letters: Minnie and me against the HMO." Our experience exemplified the tendency of some insurers to celebrate premium dollars flowing into their coffers, but to resist the paying out of claims. I know you know exactly what I'm talking about.

I call the insurance program in which I enrolled Minnie when she arrived at the Residence, "RejectCare." While that's not its real name, I believe the appellation is apt.

Here's why: It sometimes took thirty to fifty percent of my time to get the HMO to shell out for the care that Minnie received at the behest of her primary care doctor.

This often involved long hours on "hold" with RejectCare and with the concerned doctors, hospitals, and therapists who legitimately wanted payment, and who felt that Minnie had to be the source of such payment.

Selecting RejectCare was one of the biggest mistakes I ever made with respect to health insurance and, because of bureaucratic rigidity and red tape, one that took me forever to undo.

The specific program, which I call RejectCare's "Geezer Plus," had been heavily advertised and promoted as an alternative to straight Medicare for seniors.

In actual practice, the HMO used any excuse it could find, and some of these were very creative, to deny payment to the doctors who ordered the services that Minnie received.

Considering my professional background, I should have known better than to choose this particular HMO, but I was trying to conserve Minnie's dwindling assets. RejectCare's premiums were the lowest in town. As usual, you get what you pay for.

The HMO's justification for many of its denials was that Minnie's primary care physician did not follow proper procedure in ordering the services. The doctor and/or the Residence was supposed to get advance approval of these orders, but sometimes this got overlooked due to the urgency of Minnie's need.

But the fact remained that Minnie didn't order the care, and I didn't order the care. It was the doctor who felt that Minnie needed the care and who was the one who ordered it. That, in my opinion, is how it should be. RejectCare's auditors, however, had a more self-serving view of the process.

So, based on this technicality, the HMO continued to deny payment whenever it thought it could get away with it, and the health care providers involved would then dun Minnie for payment. Sound familiar?

Anyone involved in a similar fight with an HMO over denial of care to a loved one will understand what it took to win these battles...but win I did, every time.

How did I do this? Well, it seems that RejectCare was violating Medicare's rules with these denials. Of course, they didn't volunteer this information. It took some research on my part to figure this out.

My point is that it's worth your time and energy to fight them. Big bucks are often involved. Don't give up. They depend on wearing you down. Be persistent. Most of the time, they'll back down when they see you won't go away.

"HOME" SWEET HOME

For decades, my career had taken me far afield from the East Coast where Minnie and Sidney spent all of their lives. Sometimes years would go by during which my family and I would only get to see my parents for short visits at six-month intervals.

One of the anticipated joys of bringing Minnie to live near me at the Residence was the chance to visit her frequently, to monitor her well being, and to rebuild a close relationship with her.

Frankly, I sometimes wondered whether my mother, who had been so loving and "together" during my developmental years, might be having emotional problems. Her highs were becoming very high, and her lows were cycling ever deeper and more frequent. But it was a touchy subject and I am not a mental health professional.

During the period just before Sidney died, Minnie became overtly judgmental of almost everyone in her circle. Nobody seemed to measure up to what she expected of him or her—not even me, and definitely not Nadine.

"Jerry," Minnie would say, "I want to talk to you about Nadine."

"What about this time, Ma?"

"She's a wonderful girl and I know you love her..."

"But?"

"No 'buts.'"

"So what did you want to talk about?"

"She's too lenient with the kids."

"Not that again, Ma."

"You don't have to listen to me, but I do know something about raising children. Jerry, they're being spoiled."

"What do you mean?" I asked, temper flaring. "Be specific."

"I don't want to fight with you. I just think you should do something about it."

Again. "Be specific, Ma. Because I don't know what you are talking about."

"Okay. They're very hard on clothes."

"Ma, they're kids. They play ball. They ride bikes. They wrestle on the floor."

"You never did such things."

"Ma, of course I did."

"No you didn't. Your father would never have allowed it."

"I'm ending this conversation now, Ma."

"Okay, but don't come crying to me when you spend a fortune replacing their clothes."

And so it went. Early stage dementia never even occurred to me.

Her outspoken statements were driving many of her friends and even her relatives away from her. She seemed bitter and unhappy, and her conversation was filled obsessively with her perceptions about hurts, real and imagined, that happened decades before.

On the other hand, it seemed to me that much of Minnie's unhappiness was self-inflicted. I became more and more convinced that it was something that might be responsive to professional counseling.

When I finally got up my courage to suggest this to her, I was surprised to find her agreeable. The problem was Sidney.

"Jerry," he said, "why are you putting these ideas into your mother's head? Don't I have enough problems? Aren't I entitled to a little peace?"

"Dad, Mom is so unhappy lately. Haven't you noticed?"

"Of course I've noticed. But it's nothing that couldn't be fixed by having you and the kids move to Florida."

"Sorry, Dad. You know I wish we could—but I have to live where I can work. As Aunt Charlotte says, 'Home is where you make a living.'"

"I know, I know. It's just that I wish it were possible. That's all it would take to fix up your mother."

"I don't think so. I think she could use some professional help. Listen, Dad, there's no shame in it. Everyone could benefit from a bit of counseling. Even you and me. And she seems to want it."

"Jerry, only 'nutcakes' go to psychiatrists. No wife of mine is going to a shrink. Yes, Minnie is unhappy and, yes, she's driving me crazy with her behavior, but that's just her personality. She's always been this way. Forget about it!"

Surprisingly, Minnie fought him on this and insisted on getting counseling. She even had a few sessions. However, when the doctor asked for Sidney to attend too that was it. It was over.

In retrospect, Minnie's conduct at the time may well have been signaling the beginnings of her dementia. Or it might have been some other neurotic condition that could have been relieved with proper care. But we were never to know. My father stopped it cold.

So, Minnie and Sidney stayed in Florida and I continued to live in the Midwest. Sidney died and the years rolled by.

But that was all in the past. With her living nearby during the end years of her life, I hoped to make it up to her. She would be able to see some of her grandchildren much more often than ever before, and now there were great-grandchildren too.

Instead of a brief telephone contact on holidays and on family occasions Minnie, I thought, could be a participant. She could come to our home for regular family get-togethers, Sunday dinners, celebrations.

She could join us at our Synagogue for services, especially on major holidays. She could accompany us to restaurants and to see the sights in our region. It was a grand vision and, for a year or so, it actually worked out as planned.

However, it was not to last. Her dementia and her physical problems quickly limited her activities.

Among other things, I began to get monthly bills in excess of $500 for Minnie's pharmaceuticals. Here's an example of a bill for a typical month: December 2000 (whatever year it happens to be when you are reading this, rest assured that the prices will be much higher).

- Risperdal (psychotic disorders): $ 69
- Lasix (water retention): $3
- Aricept (dementia): $112
- Duratuss G (expectorant): $30
- K-Dur (potassium replacement): $25
- Celexa (antidepressant): $55
- Ditropan (genitourinary relaxant): $76
- Metamucil (regularity): $7
- Atrovent (obstructive lung disease): $35
- Serevent (asthma): $61
- Azmacort (lung spasm conditions): $49
- Tylenol Extra Strength: $7
- Levaquin (antibiotic): $74
- Singulair (chronic asthma) $33

Total Cost-Fourteen drugs: $636

Insurance covered none of it, but Minnie seemed healthy and, more important, she was happy at last. So what could I do except smile and pay, and hope she would not run out of money?

Amazingly, she did not have undesirable side effects from this regimen. Even more amazingly, she was truly a changed person. Minnie seemed happier than I could ever remember her being. So why mess with success?

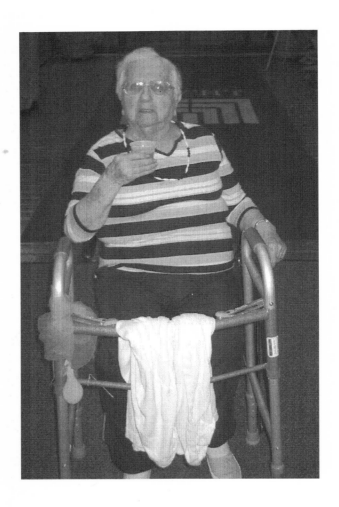

If the psychotropic medications made such a difference in her mood and temperament, my only regret was that Sidney prevented her from starting such therapy years ago. She could have enjoyed all that additional time free from her resentments and anger.

Also, her memory was getting noticeably weaker. If she used to carry a grudge for decades, and if she used to dwell obsessively on all the terrible things she believed her dearest friends and relatives had done to her, she did so no longer. She somehow became a contented person, and one who was much more pleasant to be with.

I seriously worried that Minnie's old tendency to alienate people would result in complaints from the administration of the Residence. I even feared that she might be asked to leave.

Not to worry. Staff, residents, volunteers, in fact everyone at the Residence soon were stopping me in the halls to sing my mother's praises.

"Ma, everyone loves you here."

"I like it here too. How long am I staying?"

"This is your home now. No more moves. Is that okay with you?"

"I guess so. But when am I going back to my real home?"

"Where do you think your 'real' home is?"

Silence. Then, "I don't know."

"Ma, believe me, this is where you live now."

"Thanks for telling me. I didn't know. Everyone is very nice here."

"I'm glad you like it, Ma. Do you miss Florida very much?

"I can't remember it, honey. Tell me about it."

"Well, Ma, it's where you and Dad lived together for twenty years, after you both retired, and until he died."

"Tell me again how he died. I can't remember."

"You really can't remember that?"

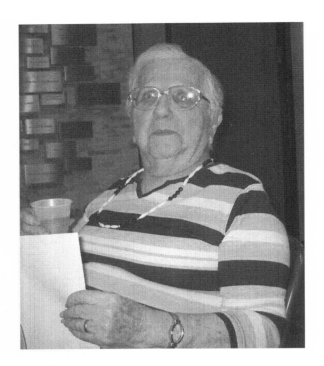

"I have 'short-term memory loss.' You have to keep telling me these things."

"You don't seem upset about having short-term memory loss."

"I'm not upset. Every day is a new day. It's kind of nice. I'm always having surprises..."

"And you can't remember the things that used to aggravate you. Right?"

"Right."

It may not be such a terrible thing to have short-term memory loss.

LONGEVITY

Dementia Diary

Minnie lived at the Residence for almost eight years before moving on to a nursing home in April 2005 at age ninety-one (more about that later).

Born in 1913, she was eighty-three when she arrived at the Residence. For a long time, she did not remember her age unless someone prompted her.

Today, even prompting gets no response." Jerry," she used to say, back when she could still hold a conversation, "I have nine lives."

"Are you a cat then, Ma? If you started with nine lives, you must have used some of them when you were hospitalized in Florida, and again up here?"

"I still have some left, Jerry. I have longevity."

"That's wonderful, Ma. But how do you know?"

"Don't worry. I know.

And she does have longevity. If she had stayed in Florida, I believe that she would not have lasted this long. She was deteriorating rapidly there. Here, she has begun the tenth decade of her life.

She is quite frail, physically, and her dementia is very pronounced, but she is very much alive. I don't know how to measure happiness in someone so near the end of a fifteen-plus year slide into total physical and cognitive dependence.

For years, in spite of her situation, she seemed happy. Now, she suffers from all sorts of new ailments. It must be hard for her to be cheerful. Still, she tries.

When I think about how long it has been since my mother was completely herself—how long she has lived in the margins of life—I am amazed. For me, bearing witness and trying to do what's right as a loving caregiver, it has been a long, slow, torturous decline.

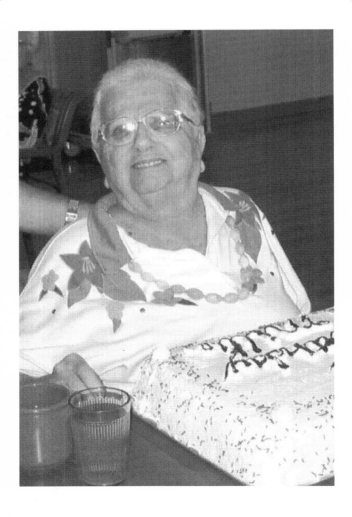

Since she cannot express herself, I can only try to imagine what it's been like for her.

When Minnie first arrived up north, we bought her new winter clothes and took her out frequently on family excursions. She loved going for Chinese food, or sharing a Sunday afternoon at our home, or going to services at our synagogue. Sadly, these things became impractical much too quickly.

Shortly after she got here, we took her to a special holiday dinner at the synagogue. We sat at a large round table with seven other people, none of whom we knew prior to that evening.

As is customary at such occasions, everyone introduced him or herself and made ongoing small talk throughout the meal. Everyone except Minnie, that is.

She was mostly silent, and she busily occupied herself by shoveling edible things onto her plate. Most folks were delaying eating until after the blessing over the bread, and I tried to get Minnie to do the same.

It was no use. She was power grazing on rolls and relishes, salad and celery sticks, in quantities that would have left me stuffed and unable to eat the entrée.

"When do I get my dinner?" she asked when the rolls were gone. "I'm hungry and I didn't even get a roll. Jerry, see if you can get the waiter to bring me a roll."

"Ma, you had three rolls already."

Angry voice, much too loud. "No I didn't!"

Heads turned.

"Yes you did. I watched you. Look at the crumbs on your bread plate. Where did those come from?"

She looked, she scowled, and she said, "I don't know, but I didn't have a roll yet, so it's not from me."

"Okay, Ma. Let's forget about it. I'll get you a roll." And I did. And she ate it.

When the entrée was served. She wolfed it down and said, "I'm still hungry, Jerry. I didn't have a roll. The waiter forgot me. Can you get me one?"

Then, loudly, referring to a woman about her age across the table that was having some trouble cutting her prime rib, "Look at her. The way she eats. Disgusting. Why do they take such people out in public?"

This is the old Minnie, I thought. She's still in there somewhere, dementia or not. But all I could say was, "Shhhh!" as my eyes darted furtively around the table to see if anyone had heard her. They had.

When the meal ended, everyone seemed relieved. I certainly was. I rushed her back to the Residence and, call me coward, that was the last outside meal that I ever took her to, other than private family functions.

The experts tell me that aged people tend to say what's on their minds. The word the social workers use for that is "disinhibited." The trouble was that if Minnie was disinhibited, the process had probably started in her teens.

This was nothing new. It was only getting worse. Some geriatric researchers have said that people don't really change in old age, but that quirks and foibles that were minor parts of their lifetime characters can become greatly exaggerated with dementia. I can vouch for that.

Months later, we had a house full of family members for our Passover Seder. They came from near and far. Minnie sat between her sister Charlotte and Charlotte's daughter, Noreen, a woman in her forties. Minnie had known and loved her niece, Noreen, since she was a little girl.

As I drove Minnie back to the Residence after the Seder, she asked, "Who was that woman sitting next to me?"

"You mean Charlotte?"

"Of course not. The one on the other side."

"Ma, that was Charlotte's daughter, your niece Noreen. Didn't you recognize her?"

"When did she get to be so old? I remember a little girl. That was a grown woman."

My heart sank. I was shocked that Minnie was unable to recognize her own niece, a woman that she had seen as an adult many times.

Even with my natural inclination toward denial, it was getting difficult to pretend that Minnie was stable. She was clearly sinking ever deeper into her daze.

Dementia Diary

LATE STAGE
DEMENTIA

Often, when Minnie was still able to make phone calls, she would do it repetitively, and she would forget that she had done so.

Once, coming home from an evening out, I checked the voicemail and found nine calls from Minnie. She was in a desperate state. You would have thought she had broken a hip or something.

The reason for her panic: the battery in her watch had stopped. I called her immediately.

"Ma," I said. "I just got home and there were nine messages from you about your watch."

"Nine messages? Jerry, I wouldn't do that. Why do you say such things?"

I was tempted to say, "Don't you remember making the calls?" However, the professionals keep telling me that phrases like "don't you remember?" or "do you recall?" are potentially hurtful to people with dementia.

Most of the time they won't remember, will be upset about being told that they did or experienced things that they can't recall and, actually, they might even pretend that they do remember.

All in all, not a good thing. It takes constant vigilance for me to stop myself from testing Minnie's memory in this way. This time, though, I was successful.

"Okay, Ma," I said. "It doesn't matter. Can you do without a watch for a few days until I can get yours fixed?"

Very agitated now. Yelling. Almost crying. "No! I must be able to tell the time. You have to do it now."

"Ma. There's a clock radio in your room, and wall clocks all over the place."

"I need my watch. I need you to fix my watch."

"Okay, okay. But it's 9:30 at night. Can't it wait till morning?"

You know what happened, don't you? A trip to the 24-hour discount store was unavoidable. However, the good news is that it solved the problem.

Having her watch working again calmed Minnie down, so we all could get some sleep.

The irony is that she stopped wearing it a few months later.

"Ma. You're not wearing your watch."

"I don't think I have one."

"You do and I know where it is. Do you want me to get it?"

"No. I don't need it."

She was in a different place, cognitively speaking. Since she could no longer make phone calls, for several years I called her. Every day. From wherever in the world I happened to be.

She loved these calls, even if she couldn't remember them the next day. Then she lost the ability to hang up the phone and I had to stop calling her.

She could no longer find her way to her room, the nursing station, the dining room, or anyplace else in the Residence without someone's guidance.

If they changed the décor of a common room and set it up for a party, she thought she was in another building.

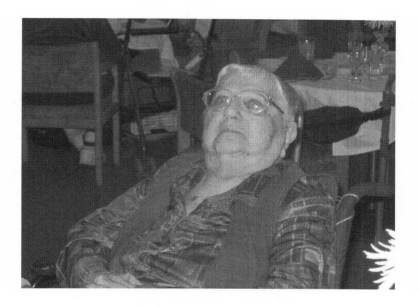

On one such occasion, after the meal, I said, "The party's over, Ma. Let me help you back to your room."

"Okay. Go get the car and I'll be ready."

"Why the car? Your room is upstairs."

"It is?" Laughing. "I get so mixed up. You mean I'm already home."

"You are. This is your regular dining room. It just looks different because of the party decorations."

"Really? I didn't know. Thanks for telling me."

If one talked to her, she responded with what the professionals call "empty speech."

"How are you, Ma?"

"Fine"

"There's a movie in the club room. Do you want to go?"

"I love you." She blows a kiss.

"What about the movie?"

"What movie?"

"The one in the clubroom."

"There's a movie in the clubroom?"

"Yes. You'll love it. It's an oldie with Jimmie Stewart."

"I love Jimmy Stewart."

"I know. Want to go?"

"Go where?"

"The movie in the clubroom?"

"No."

Today, Minnie no longer reads or watches TV. Her attention span is too short. For about a year, Minnie spent several days each week in a day care program for people with dementia. It is physically attached to the Residence.

This was a fabulous addition to her life. Even though she lost her ability to initiate anything, she was kept busy and stimulated, and she enjoyed interacting with the other clients.

During Minnie's admission interview for this program, I had to answer most of the questions. Minnie could not say the date of her birthday or her correct age. She could not identify America's current President, the correct day of the week, or provide other basic information. She tried guessing, but was way off on most questions.

With me, her only child, sitting there, the social worker asked, "Mrs. Sweet, how many children do you have?"

Without hesitating, Minnie replied, "Two, I think."

At first, I was stunned. "Ma," I said. "You always said I was your only child."

She looked at me and started to laugh. "That's true," she said through her mirth.

"Do I have any brothers or sisters I don't know about?" I asked, wondering if that might be so.

"No. I don't know why I said two. You're the only one."

The social worker looked puzzled, joined in the laughter, and asked, "So, how many is it?"

"Put down 'one'," I said.

Usually, when I visited Minnie those days, I found her sitting and sleeping in the lobby, just like those residents she scrutinized negatively on the day she was admitted. But she didn't remember being disturbed by the sight, and she didn't express any bad feelings about having become one of "them."

"Hello, Ma," I would say, waking her up. Her eyes would open and her face light up.

"What are you doing here?"

"I came to see you. Did I wake you?"

"I wasn't sleeping."

"How are you feeling?"

"Fine, now that you are here." She blows a kiss. "You don't come enough."

"I was here two days ago."

Smiles. "Thanks for telling me."

"How's your back pain?"

"It doesn't hurt. They give me Tylenol."

"And your breathing?"

"It's good."

"Do you still get breathing treatments?"

"I think so."

"It's a lovely day today. Want to go outside and sit awhile."

"No. My back hurts and I have trouble breathing."

"You just told me these things weren't bothering you."

"I did?"

"Yes. So your back is hurting. Let me ask the nurse for some Tylenol."

"What for?"

"For your back pain."

"My back doesn't hurt."

And so it usually goes.

There was still humor in Minnie's life at this point, and the ability for her to laugh at herself. Her laughter was not self-demeaning, but affectionate. Here are some examples.

Minnie's mealtimes were taken during the second seating. Her lunch was usually at 12:30, so I sometimes visited at 11:30.

On one such visit, I couldn't find her. I looked in her room, in the activity rooms, at the nursing station, in the beauty parlor, and even asked an Aide to check the bathrooms. No Minnie.

Finally, the dietary staff said she was eating lunch during the first seating. They said she claimed to be very hungry, so they made an unusual exception and let her get seated early. I found her in the dining room at a table with two other residents, a man and a woman.

"Ma," I said. "I couldn't find you. I looked everywhere. How come you are eating early?"

"I don't know. They just started serving me."

"They told me you said you were hungry."

"Nah! Let me get up. I'll eat later."

"No, that's alright. You have a plate of lunch in front of you. I don't want to disturb you. I'll see you again in two days."

At this point, the other woman at the table jumped in. "Who is this lady to you?" she asked. "Your aunt...your sister...who?"

"She's my mother."

"Your mother? And you are leaving? Listen, If she's your mother you have to be much more attentive."

"Yeah," chimed in the man at the table. "I didn't see you kiss her."

"I didn't see you kiss her, either," I replied, and everyone had a good laugh including Minnie, whose wide smile revealed something I hadn't noticed before.

"Ma, where are your teeth?"

She opened her mouth wide and pointed to her lower dentures.

"Ma, what about your upper dentures?"

"What about them?"

"They're missing."

"They are?" She said touching her upper gums. "Oh, they are!" And she started to laugh. "That's funny," she said.

"Ma, how are you eating without your uppers?"

"I don't know. I didn't know they were gone. I was eating okay."

A frantic search by the staff eventually turned up Minnie's teeth in her laundry, to everyone's relief and amusement. A big expense and major hassle avoided. That time.

Another anecdote. Nadine and I were in Los Angeles waiting in a line of cars to enter the Getty Museum. As we reached the fee booth before the parking facility my cell phone rang. It was the nurse at the Residence over 2000 miles away.

"You'd better come back immediately," she said. "She's had a serious setback, will not get out of bed, eat, or take her medicines. We don't think she'll ever get out of bed again."

Talk about stress. "I have a flight back in 3 hours," I said as the woman in the booth held out her hand for the entry fee. What am I doing here, I thought, "Will I make it on time?" I said to the nurse.

"That's hard to say. Try to get here as soon as you can."

My heart falling, I called my son who lived near Minnie. He dropped everything and went immediately to the Residence."

"It looks pretty grave," he said when he called back. "Hurry home."

So it was a tense and terrifying ten hours that followed. All the way home, Nadine and I wondered if we'd make it on time. When we finally approached the Residence in our car, I said, "I'm not sure I can handle this. I mean, what will we find inside? Will Mom be alive or dying or, God forbid, already gone? Nadine, I don't want to find out."

Expecting the worst, we timidly entered the Memory Unit. Guess what? Minnie was up and seated at a table in the dining room. When she saw us, she smiled and waved with great energy.

"Hi," she said. "How are ya?" She showed no signs of the deathwatch we anticipated, nor did she have any memory of what happened.

"She's amazing, your mother," the nurse said. "She did another one of her 180's."

Do I need to describe my emotions at that moment? I think not.

The fallout though, was a decision by all concerned, to arrange for Minnie to apply to a hospice for special services to patients nearing death and their families. One look by the hospice doctor and Minnie was accepted into their program.

So I was on official notice. The professionals thought Minnie would soon be dead. What an emotional roller coaster! I was going from laughter to tears and back again faster than the speed of light.

Dementia Diary

PERPETUAL EMOTION

Gradually, Minnie's ability to walk more than a few yards without a rest was curtailed by her growing respiratory problems. She would gasp for breath, be unable to speak, and would need to sit down many times before reaching her destination. It could take ten minutes for her to go a hundred feet.

Several nasty falls landed her in the emergency rooms of local hospitals, and rewarded her with the walker she had dreaded so much—but her attitude had changed. She actually loved her walker. She really needed it, was afraid to walk without it, and could not recall her prior revulsion at the thought of it.

As I write this, it is several years later and she is now wheelchair bound. I remember her walker with nostalgia. She was slow, but at least she could get around on her own.

Also, she is totally incontinent. At first it was just her bladder. With the persuasive efforts of the social work staff, Minnie reluctantly agreed to wear protective underwear. For about a year, that did the trick. She was able to self-toilet and she could still go almost anywhere.

After a while she gave up self-toileting altogether. She would often leave damp spots on chairs when she arose, and her pants would be visibly wet. Remarkably, she seemed unaware of this, but I still felt embarrassed for her. I worried a lot about protecting her dignity.

Eventually, she lost total control of her bowels too, and fully absorbent diapers had to be introduced. She no longer resisted this. By this time, her personal hygiene required frequent changes and showers each day.

Something must happen to the sense of smell and tactile sensitivity in late stage dementia. Minnie never knows when she has a diaper full until one of her personal care aides peeks and takes her to her room for clean up. You would think she'd feel uncomfortable, or notice the odor, or be embarrassed. But she seems oblivious.

How do I feel about this? How is a son supposed to feel? We're talking about the woman who lovingly toilet-trained me.

When I see her like this, I feel like the contents of those dirty diapers. My feelings bounce up and down like a basketball keeping pace with Minnie's changing personality and deficiencies. They range between highs of love and respect and lows of resentment and frustration.

Mostly, there is just heartbreak at witnessing this once vital and intelligent woman lose herself within her own failing body.

As you might expect, all of Minnie's breathing, walking, and toileting issues made it very difficult for me to handle her needs. Under these conditions, outside excursions had to taper off, and eventually they stopped altogether. I still mourn their loss.

From Minnie's perspective, however, the absence of such jaunts never became an issue. She never once said, "How come you don't take me out anymore?" There were plenty of things to entertain her when she lived at the Residence.

Something special happens every day at the Residence. There are musical presentations, group low-impact exercises, a garden club, jewelry making, current events and other lectures, movies, holiday celebrations, visits from schoolchildren, bingo (of course), fashion shows, birthday parties, and on and on and on. It's endless stimulation.

For the first four or five years, Minnie was an active participant in all these events. Drawing on her background as a community organizer, she attended meetings of the Resident Council, started conversations, kept track of the schedule of events, got herself to activities without reminding, knew where she was "geographically" in the building, easily found her way to her room, socialized with other residents, made phone calls, asked questions of me and staff, and otherwise made her presence felt.

This is no longer true.

At first, too, Minnie was a frequent user of the well-stocked library at the Residence—but failing eyesight and cognition soon prevented her from reading—and she lost the strength in her hands to hold a book.

As she declined, Minnie was fortunate to be accepted into a new day care program for the memory impaired and, later, into a dedicated residential program for people with Alzheimer's disease or other dementias.

I hoped she could eventually end her days in the comfort of these familiar and supportive surroundings. In fact, every effort was made by staff and management to help my mother to age in place—and for this I am truly grateful.

Minnie, however, eventually lost the ability to take advantage of the program on the Memory Unit. She could sometimes respond to a direct question or stimulant, but she could no longer initiate conversation or action, or participate in the structured Unit activities.

It soon became obvious that Minnie's dementia had reached the point where the Memory Unit could not help her. Clearly, someone on the waiting list, less severely impaired than Minnie, would be able to utilize these services more effectively. So I did what she begged me ten years previously never to do. I "put her" in a nursing home.

I won't go into the pain and horror of shopping for, evaluating, choosing, and paying for a nursing home. There are many good books already available that can help a family with that task (e.g. "Choosing A Nursing Home" by Dr. Seth B. Goldsmith, Prentice Hall Press).

I'll only say that there are few fabulous nursing homes out there. Again, we got lucky and found a facility that, on balance, provides reasonably acceptable care. So she was admitted.

How did Minnie react to her move to the dreaded nursing home?

"Ma," I asked, the day after the move. "How do you like your new home?"

She looked around, then at me, and she smiled and shrugged as if to say, "What new home?"

Rather than answer directly, I asked another loaded question about her new living arrangement, something I felt guilty about.

She had gone from an almost private room to the center bed of a three bed room, the only dividers being thin, hospital type curtains—and one of her roommates moaned and groaned continuously far into the night.

"Ma," I asked. "Are you okay with your new room?"

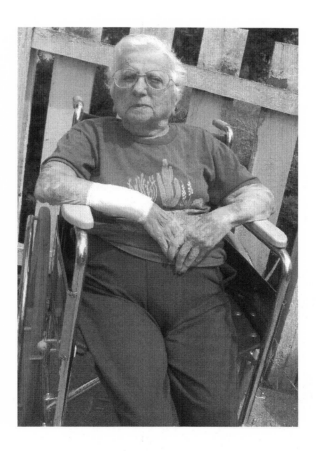

Again she shrugged. She tried to say, "What new room?"—but she wasn't able to complete the sentence.

I ignored that too and asked, "Are you being annoyed or kept awake by your roommate's noises?"

Conveniently, the roommate let out a loud shriek at that moment. If Minnie heard it, you'd never know from her demeanor. She looked at me with a bewildered stare and quietly shook her head.

A new phase had begun.

***

There are literally dozens of anecdotes that I could add to this narrative. Yet, it strikes me that this is as good a place as any to end the tale.

Earlier in this book, I described the stress associated with Minnie's relocation up north, and why I tried to resist bringing her to live near me. Yet, with good, clear hindsight, there is no question that it was the right thing to do.

As a male caregiver, with no siblings, and with a family, a business, and a life of my own, I shudder at what these years would have been like had I allowed Minnie to remain in Florida. I cannot imagine how I would have coped long distance with the daily challenges associated with her deepening dementia.

Also, I never would have known the satisfaction I have experienced in sharing Minnie's last years in the manner described. She and I have enjoyed a treasured period during which past irritations have been set aside and only gentleness and tenderness remains.

Whatever happens next, we have had this boon.

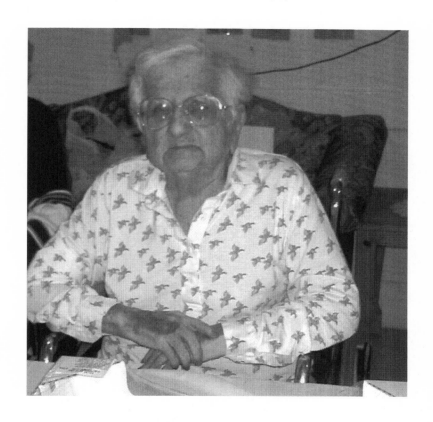

Her 92nd Birthday
September 2005

BOOKEND—2003

"Only poetry can measure the distance between ourselves and the Other."

—*Charles Simic*

The truth is that she did not die
She was not ready to say goodbye
But like a fairy butterfly
She makes me face the truth

From her cocoon she struggled out
Not knowing what her life's about
Too frail to rage and rant and shout
She makes me face the truth

She's gentle now...her anger gone
She's sweet and kind—a paragon
Who's loved and praised by everyone
She makes me face the truth

Her memory is very weak
As is her shrunken bent physique
Her voice is raspy...when she speaks
She makes me face the truth

She can't recall her family
And friends she knew will ever be
Gone…forgotten…absentee
She makes me face the truth

The truth is that I miss the days
She made me crazy with her ways
This cheery cherub's face portrays
A stranger's unknown truth

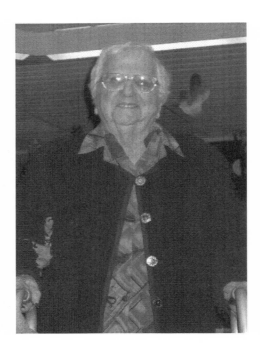

2003

Dementia Diary

ABOUT THE AUTHOR

Robert Tell (AKA Jerry Sweet) is a writer who lives near his Mom in Farmington Hills, Michigan. He was born and raised in Brooklyn, New York and educated in Public Health and English at Columbia and Long Island Universities. He nourished his creative writing habit while working as a hospital administrator, health planning agency executive, health policy professor, and business owner.

Bob's poetry, columns, articles, and creative non-fiction have appeared in many periodicals, including *The World and I, Mediphors, Arts Borealis, PKA's Advocate, Peninsula Poets, Northeast Outdoors, Detroit Jewish News,* Detroit's *Health Care Weekly Review, Hospitals JAHA, Modern Hospital, Hospital and Health Services Administration, Journal of the American College of Emergency Physicians,* and two *United Nations* sponsored anthologies.

Just like his parents before him, Bob and his wife, Elaine, snowbird each winter to Southeastern Florida. His adult children and his incredibly talented grandchildren live in the Seattle, San Francisco and Ann Arbor areas. This gives him lots of great places to visit.

.

Made in the USA
Lexington, KY
06 January 2012